FATTY LIVER DIET

COOKBOOK FOR BEGINNERS

Explore A Collection Of Mouthwatering Recipes Tailored For Liver Health, Crafted To Support Your Well-Being While Satisfying Your Taste Buds

JESSICA C. STEPHEN

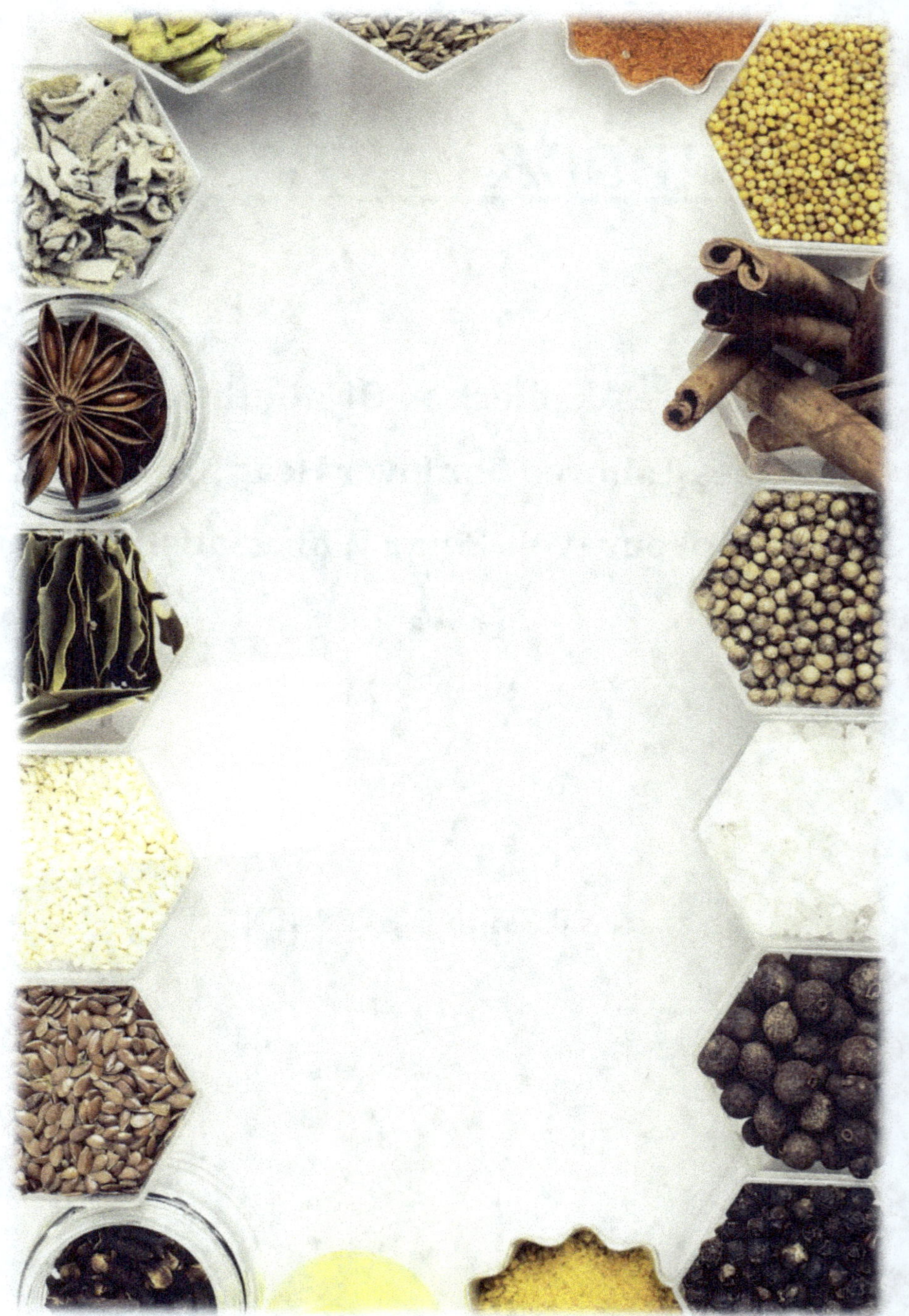

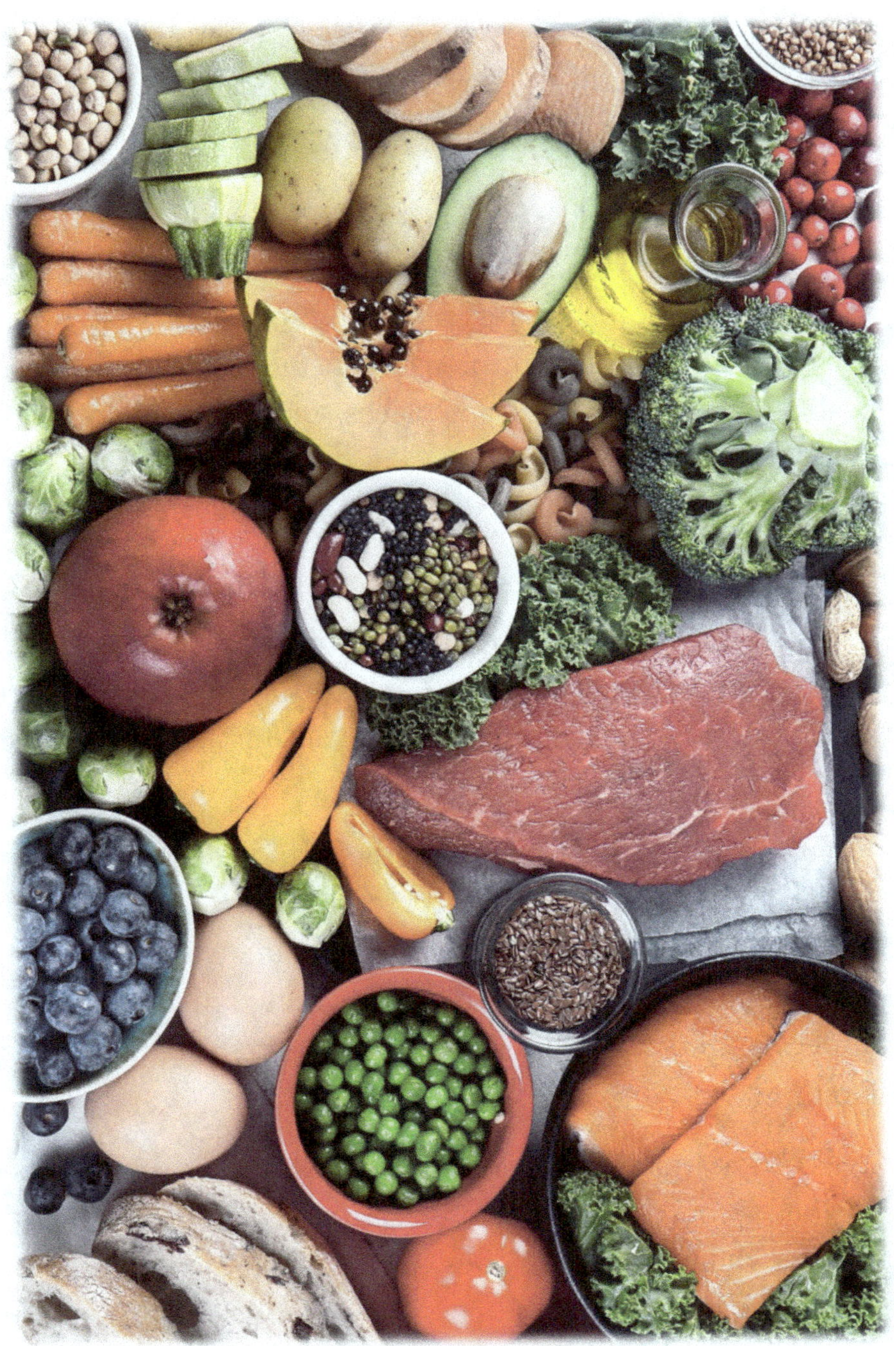

Disclaimer

The information in this book is meant solely for educational reasons. This book's contents are not meant to be used in place of expert medical advice, diagnosis, or treatment. Any decisions you make about your health must be discussed with a licensed healthcare provider.

Every effort has been made by the author to guarantee that the material in this book is correct and current as of the date of publication. Still, since medical knowledge advances rapidly, new studies might be conducted that change our understanding this illness and how best to manage it with food.

This book may contains references to and mentions of various people, things, websites, organizations, and other entities that the author does not support, advocate, or have any association with. There is no implied sponsorship or collaboration; all references and remarks are made only for informational purposes.

In order to address their individual health concerns, readers are advised to independently verify any information contained in this book and to consult with healthcare specialists. Any negative effects arising from the use or implementation of the material in this book, whether direct or indirect, are not the responsibility of the author or the publisher.

The dietary suggestions and counsel provided in this book are broad in scope and might not be appropriate for every individual. Readers are recommended to seek tailored counsel from trained healthcare specialists as individual health problems and demands differ.

The reader accepts the conditions of this disclaimer by reading this book.

FACTS ABOUT THIS BOOK

The book "Liver Health diet cookbook" is essential in enlightening people about the vital relationship between diet and liver health. The introduction offers a thorough explanation of the significance of liver health, illuminating prevalent liver disorders and highlighting the role of diet in preserving ideal liver function. It is a priceless tool for anyone looking to improve the health of their liver through food.

The book's comprehensive approach is exemplified by the table of contents, which covers the vital vitamins, minerals, and nutrients that are critical for liver health. The book's dedication to offering a comprehensive grasp of nutritional components crucial for liver function is demonstrated by the inclusion of recipes high in vitamins A, C, and E as well as information on the significance of B vitamins, selenium, and zinc.

The book's emphasis on doable and tasty dishes that support liver function is one of its key features.

The recipes, which include high-fiber foods, lean protein sources, and omega-3 fatty acids, are designed to promote detoxification and digestive health. There are recipes for water-infused drinks and detoxifying herbal teas that underscore the importance of staying hydrated while undergoing a liver detox.

In addition, the book discusses how blood sugar levels affect liver function and provides low-glycemic index cooking options. It offers a well-rounded method of meal planning that includes whole grains, beans, and sugary foods with low blood sugar impact. Colorful fruit and vegetable salads are featured in the section on meals high in antioxidants, which promotes a diet high in preventive components.

The book also reaches out to people with special dietary requirements by providing liver-friendly recipes for vegetarians and people on restricted diets. Discussing the effects of processed foods on liver health, offering substitutes, and highlighting the significance of reading labels, encourages consumers to make educated decisions.

This book is a comprehensive resource because it includes lifestyle advice for liver health, including the importance of exercise, stress reduction techniques, and other lifestyle modifications. Weekly meal plans, advice on batch cooking, and support for sustainable lifestyle modifications provide people with useful resources to incorporate liver-friendly habits into their everyday lives.

Finally, "Liver Health Recipes" is unique in that it is a thorough manual that extends beyond recipes. It informs readers about the significance of liver health, offers a wide range of delectable and nourishing recipes, and gives helpful lifestyle advice for long-term well-being. This book is an invaluable tool for anyone trying to prioritize and improve liver health, whether they are working to prevent liver diseases or manage ones that already exist.

Table of Contents

CHAPTER 1

OVERVIEW OF LIVER HEALTH

Recognizing The Significance Of Liver Health

The liver is an essential organ that serves a variety of purposes that are essential to preserving general health. It functions as a metabolic engine and is essential for nutrient storage, cleansing, and digesting. Considering the liver's involvement in numerous physiological processes, it is imperative to comprehend the significance of liver health. The liver helps with blood glucose regulation, bile production for digestion, and the breakdown of nutrients from the food we eat. It additionally removes pollutants from the bloodstream and functions as a detoxifying agent.

The liver is not indestructible, though, and several things can harm or deteriorate the liver. The liver can be strained by lifestyle decisions such as binge drinking enormous amounts of alcohol, eating a diet heavy in processed foods, and being sedentary.

The health of the liver may also be threatened by hereditary disorders, certain drugs, and viral diseases like hepatitis. Adopting behaviors that protect the liver begins with acknowledging how important it is to keep it in good health.

Typical Liver Disorders

Its functionality can be compromised by several liver disorders, underscoring the importance of taking preventative health measures. The liver becomes inflamed when someone has hepatitis, which can be brought on by infections, excessive alcohol consumption, or autoimmune diseases. Another common illness is non-alcoholic fatty liver disease (NAFLD), which is frequently associated with obesity and insulin resistance. Prolonged liver injury can lead to cirrhosis, a late stage of liver tissue scarring.

A serious outcome of long-term liver ailments, liver cancer is frequently linked to underlying illnesses like cirrhosis. Alcoholic liver disease, which results from long-term alcohol misuse, can show up as cirrhosis, alcoholic hepatitis, or fatty liver. Early intervention and successful management of several common liver disorders depend on the ability to recognize their signs and symptoms.

Nutrition's Function in the Liver

Maintaining healthy liver function and preventing liver disorders are greatly aided by proper nutrition. The maintenance of liver health requires a diet that is well-balanced and rich in a range of nutrients. Fruits and vegetables, which are high in antioxidants, aid in the fight against oxidative stress and liver inflammation. Nuts and avocados are good sources of healthy fats that promote bile synthesis and liver function in general.

Appropriate protein consumption is necessary for the repair and regeneration of tissue, which are vital processes for a healthy liver. Fat buildup in the liver can be avoided by consuming fewer processed meals, sweetened beverages, and saturated fats. Sufficient hydration is also essential for supporting different metabolic processes and eliminating pollutants.

In summary, fostering a healthy liver requires adopting a nutritionally sound diet, realizing the significance of liver health, and identifying common liver problems. People can prevent liver disorders and improve their overall health by leading a lifestyle that promotes liver health.

CHAPTER 2

CRUCIAL ELEMENTS FOR A HEALTHY LIVER

<u>Rich In Vitamins A, C, And E Recipes</u>

Vitamins A, C, and E are essential for maintaining the health and function of the liver. These vital minerals fight oxidative stress and liver inflammation by acting as potent antioxidants. Recipes high in these vitamins shield the liver from harm brought on by free radicals, improving liver health generally.

Foods high in vitamin A, such as spinach, carrots, and sweet potatoes, help the liver remove toxic chemicals from the body. It contributes to the synthesis of bile, a digestive juice that is essential for the breakdown of lipids. Furthermore, vitamin A prevents the deterioration of liver cells by preserving their integrity.

Citrus fruits, strawberries, and bell peppers are rich sources of vitamin C, which is well-known for strengthening the immune system. Regarding liver health, vitamin C increases the body's synthesis of glutathione, an effective antioxidant that supports the body's detoxification systems. Additionally protecting liver cells from harm, this vitamin aids in the renewal of other antioxidants.

Nuts, seeds, and vegetable oils are good sources of vitamin E, another antioxidant that shields liver cells from oxidative damage. Enzymes that aid in detoxification are encouraged to work properly, which helps the liver eliminate toxic chemicals. You can help maintain the health of your liver and prevent diseases like fatty liver disease by including recipes high in vitamin E in your diet.

B Vitamins' Significance For Liver Function

B vitamins are essential for maintaining liver function. These include B1 (thiamine), B2 (riboflavin), B3 (niacin), B6 (pyridoxine), B9 (folate), and B12 (cobalamin). The metabolism of proteins, lipids, and carbohydrates is just one of the metabolic processes that these water-soluble vitamins are engaged in.

To sustain healthy neuron function and turn food into energy, thiamine (B1) is necessary. The liver uses riboflavin (B2) to help with the metabolism of lipids, medications, and steroids. The synthesis of fatty acids and the creation of energy are both aided by niacin (B3). The metabolism of amino acids depends on pyridoxine (B6), while DNA synthesis and repair depend on folate (B9).

Animal products contain B12, which is essential for the production of red blood cells and the upkeep of the neurological system. B vitamin deficiencies can cause fatty liver disease and other liver-related problems, such as compromised detoxification systems.

Including a range of B vitamin-rich foods in your diet, such as leafy green vegetables, lean meats, whole grains, and legumes, can help to maintain good liver function and promote general well-being.

Including Minerals Such As Zinc And Selenium

Zinc and selenium are two important minerals that help the liver's detoxifying functions and general health. Brazil nuts, seafood, and whole grains are rich sources of selenium, which is essential for the production of antioxidant enzymes that shield the liver from oxidative damage. Additionally, it affects how thyroid hormones are metabolized, which has an indirect effect on liver function.

Zinc has a crucial role in the production of proteins and the control of immunological responses. It can be found in foods including meat, nuts, and seeds. Zinc aids in detoxification in the liver by taking part in the production of metallothionein, a protein that binds to heavy metals and makes them easier to remove from the body.

A diverse diet that provides a balanced intake of zinc and selenium enhances the liver's resistance to toxins and supports general health. Recipes that use foods high in these minerals can be a great way to add variety to a diet that is friendly to the liver and protects it from potential damage.

CHAPTER 3

FOODS GOOD FOR THE LIVER

Healthy Liver Sources Of Lean Protein

Using lean protein sources is one of the main components of liver-friendly recipes. Proteins are necessary to sustain liver function and are also vital for sustaining general health. Choosing lean protein sources is essential for liver health since they have less saturated fat, which lessens the strain on the liver.

Fish is a great option, especially omega-3 fatty acid-rich varieties like trout, salmon, and mackerel. These fats have anti-inflammatory qualities that help the liver in addition to supporting a healthy cardiovascular system. Lean meats like turkey or chicken breast, skinless chicken, and plant-based protein sources like tofu and lentils are also excellent choices for adding lean proteins to liver-friendly dishes.

Lean proteins reduce stress on the liver and promote regeneration and repair of the organ. They supply the amino acids required for the synthesis of proteins and enzymes essential to liver function. A well-rounded nutritional approach to maintaining liver function is ensured when a range of these lean protein sources are used in recipes for liver health.

High-Fibre Foods With Liver-Friendly Recipes For Digestive Health

Fiber is essential for maintaining digestive health, and it can be especially helpful to include foods high in fiber in recipes that are good for the liver. In addition to reducing constipation and encouraging the growth of good gut flora, fiber also helps maintain a healthy weight, both of which are important for the function of the liver as a whole.

Any diet that is high in fiber and beneficial to the liver should start with fruits and vegetables. Excellent options include leafy greens, cruciferous veggies (broccoli, Brussels sprouts), and colorful fruits (apples, berries). Nuts, legumes, and whole grains are also rich in dietary fiber and can be added to meals that are suitable for the liver.

High-fiber diets affect liver health because of their capacity to control blood sugar, lower cholesterol, and promote a healthy weight. Furthermore, some meals contain soluble fiber, which functions as a prebiotic by feeding good gut bacteria that support liver and digestive health in general. Meals that taste good and actively support liver health can be made by combining a range of high-fiber foods into recipes that are liver-friendly.

Omega-3 Fatty Acids And Good Fats In Recipes For Liver Health

It is important to maintain good liver function by using healthy fats in recipes for liver health, despite the common notion that all fats are bad. There are several advantages that healthy fats, particularly those high in omega-3 fatty acids, offer for liver health.

Fish that are high in fat, such as trout, sardines, and salmon, are excellent providers of omega-3 fatty acids. The anti-inflammatory qualities of these vital fats can aid in lowering liver inflammation and enhancing liver health in general. Monounsaturated fats, which support a healthy heart and, consequently, a healthy liver, can also be found in olive oil, avocados, and nuts, which can be added to recipes that are good for the liver.Omega-3 fatty acids are essential for preserving the structural integrity and maximizing the function of liver cell membranes. They also help to avoid diseases like non-alcoholic fatty liver disease (NAFLD) by reducing the amount of fat that builds up in the liver. People can support their livers and enjoy fulfilling, savory meals that improve their general well-being by giving healthy fats priority in recipes for liver health.

CHAPTER 4

DETOXIFICATION AND HYDRATION

<u>Water's Importance In Liver Detox</u>

Staying well hydrated is essential for preserving the health of the liver and speeding up the detoxification process. One important organ in the process of removing poisons from the bloodstream is the liver. Water is necessary for these functions because it helps the liver eliminate chemicals, waste materials, and other dangerous things.

The liver may effectively remove toxins from the body through urine when the body is well-hydrated. Water serves as a medium for a variety of enzymatic activities that occur in the liver, facilitating the smooth operation of these enzymes. Furthermore, maintaining enough hydration reduces the risk of concentrated bile production, which is harmful and essential for detoxification and digestion.

It takes more than just drinking water to be hydrated when it comes to liver health. Consuming foods high in water content, such as fruits and vegetables, will help hydrate the body even more. These foods provide vital nutrients that assist liver function in addition to helping one's total fluid intake. Consequently, it is essential to keep up regular and sufficient water consumption to support liver detoxification and general well-being.

Herbal Infusions and Teas that Detoxify

It has long been known that herbal teas and infusions can aid in liver health and cleansing. Some herbs have qualities that help the liver better balance and flush out toxins from the body. Herbs including milk thistle, dandelion, and turmeric are frequently used in liver-detoxifying teas.

For example, dandelion tea is well-known for its diuretic qualities, which encourage greater urine production and help the body rid itself of pollutants.

A substance found in milk thistle called silymarin supports liver cell regeneration by acting as an antioxidant and an anti-inflammatory. Curcumin, the main ingredient in turmeric, has anti-inflammatory and antioxidant qualities that support liver function.

Herbs that are good for the liver can be included in your routine gently and naturally with these tasty herbal teas. Frequent intake of these infusions can support a healthy diet and enhance the liver's general health.

Water-Based Recipes for Clearing the Liver

Including recipes with water as part of your diet can be a tasty and revitalizing approach to aid with liver cleansing. The hydrating properties of water are combined with the tastes and nutrients of fruits, vegetables, and herbs to create infused water. Ginger, lemon, cucumber, mint, and cucumber are common additions to recipes for liver-friendly infused water.

For instance, lemon-infused water offers a dosage of vitamin C, which is necessary for the synthesis of glutathione, a potent antioxidant that is vital to the detoxification of the liver. Mint provides a refreshing touch, and cucumber adds taste and hydration. Due to its anti-inflammatory qualities, ginger can help aid in the liver's detoxification procedures.

These dishes with added water are not only tasty but also encourage people to stay hydrated regularly by consuming more fluids throughout the day. These recipes help achieve the dual objectives of supporting effective detoxification and preserving a healthy liver by making drinking more water more pleasant.

CHAPTER 5

RECIPES FOR DETOXIFICATION

<u>Juices And Smoothies For Detox</u>

In the world of liver health recipes, detox smoothies, and juices are cool drinks that help initiate the body's natural detoxification processes. These drinks usually contain a variety of nutrient-dense fruits and vegetables that are well-known for their ability to cleanse the liver. Antioxidants and vitamins found in foods like kale, spinach, beetroot, and citrus fruits aid in the liver's removal of toxins.

Beetroot is a major ingredient in these mixtures because of its high betalains content. These substances contribute to an overall detoxifying impact by helping to lower oxidative stress and inflammation in the liver. Turmeric, which is frequently praised for its strong anti-inflammatory and antioxidant qualities, also gives these detox drinks a significant boost. Turmeric curcumin is thought to benefit liver function by encouraging the generation of bile, which is necessary for detoxification and digesting.

It's important to emphasize how important it is to include high-fiber foods in these smoothies, including flaxseed and chia seeds. In addition to helping with digestion, fiber also binds to toxins and makes it easier for the body to expel them. In addition, fruit sugars naturally contain sugars that are healthier than processed sweets, so the liver won't be overworked throughout the detoxification process.

Clearing Broths And Soups

Soups and broths that are cleansing become warm, soothing partners on the path to better liver health. A variety of vegetables, herbs, and spices with detoxifying qualities are frequently used in these recipes. Broccoli and cauliflower, among other cruciferous vegetables, have chemicals in them that help the liver's detoxifying enzymes break down pollutants.

Garlic is one notable component that is commonly used in these soups. In addition to adding a strong taste, garlic is known for its sulfur-containing components, which help cleanse the liver. Studies have looked into the possibility of garlic's allicin to lessen fatty deposits and toxins' damaging effects on the liver. Another golden-hued spice that appears here is turmeric, whose curcumin content aids in its anti-inflammatory and antioxidant properties.

It's a calculated decision to add bone broth to purifying soups. Bone broth, which is high in amino acids like proline and glycine, helps the liver with its phase 2 detoxification activities. Specifically, glycine is essential for the production of glutathione, a potent antioxidant that is critical for liver function. These soups offer more than just delicious food—their nutrient-rich characteristics offer a satisfying and cleansing experience.

Veggie Bowls And Detox Salads

Vegetable bowls and detox salads are a colorful and crunchy way to support liver function. Leafy greens, lean meats, and a variety of vibrant veggies are frequently the main ingredients in these recipes. Chlorophyll, found in abundance in dark, leafy greens like kale and arugula, is thought to help the liver eliminate heavy metals and other pollutants, therefore facilitating the detoxification process.

Brussels sprouts and cabbage, two vegetables high in sulfur, are essential to the detox salad experience. Glutathione is an extremely powerful antioxidant that the liver produces, and it requires sulfur to be synthesized. Through increased production of glutathione, these veggies aid in the liver's capacity to efficiently eliminate toxins.

Avocado adds a healthy dose of monounsaturated fats to these salads, which are not only satiating but also aid in the absorption of fat-soluble vitamins, which are essential for liver function in general. The omega-3 fatty acids found in walnuts and flaxseeds, among other nuts and seeds, have anti-inflammatory qualities that help strengthen the liver's defenses against inflammation.

CHAPTER 6

LOW-GLYCEMIC INDEX RECIPES

<u>Managing Blood Sugar Levels For Liver Health</u>

For those who are worried about the health of their liver, it is essential to maintain stable blood sugar levels because blood sugar swings can directly affect liver function. Due to its ability to store and release glucose as needed, the liver is a key component in blood sugar regulation. People with liver health issues must prioritize low-glycemic index diets to avoid sudden increases in blood sugar levels. Selecting carbs that are low on the glycemic index guarantees a more gradual and regulated release of glucose into the bloodstream, avoiding excessive strain on the liver.

Blood sugar levels can only be stabilized by including a range of nutrient-dense vegetables, lean meats, and healthy fats in the diet. Meals that support liver function can include leafy greens, cruciferous vegetables, and lean proteins like fish and chicken as main ingredients. Including meals high in fiber also aids in slowing down the absorption of glucose, causing the liver to work less hard and boosting sustainable energy levels.

Moreover, controlling portion sizes is essential for maintaining blood sugar levels and liver function. It may be helpful to eat smaller, more frequent meals spaced out throughout the day to avoid sharp rises in blood sugar. This dietary pattern helps to improve metabolic health and liver function by giving the liver a consistent supply of nutrients without overloading it.

Whole Grains And Dishes Made With Legumes

The cornerstones of a low-glycemic index diet that supports liver health are whole grains and legumes. These foods, which are lower in blood sugar impact than refined carbs, include quinoa, brown rice, lentils, and beans. They are also high in fiber and other important nutrients. Because of its high fiber content, which promotes weight management—a crucial component of liver health—it helps with digestion, slows down the absorption of carbohydrates, and increases feelings of fullness.

Because whole grains include complex carbs, which release glucose gradually, they give you a steady supply of energy without spiking your blood sugar too quickly. Legumes are also a great source of plant-based proteins, which support liver health by aiding in the upkeep and repair of muscles.

Whole grains and legumes can be tasty and nutrient-dense additions to dishes. In addition to being palatable, foods like quinoa salads, lentil soups, and bean-based stews help maintain stable blood sugar levels and healthy liver function.

Sweets With Minimal Blood Sugar Impact

Even though it's well known that consuming too much sugar can harm the liver, people nevertheless have a craving for sweets. Desserts can be enjoyed without significantly raising blood sugar levels, though, if you choose low-glycemic options.

Prioritizing liver health by switching to natural sweeteners like stevia or monk fruit instead of processed sugars is a wise move. These sugar substitutes offer a gratifying sweetness without raising blood sugar levels. Furthermore, adding berries and cherries—fruits with a lower glycemic index—to sweets might improve their flavor and nutritional content.

Making desserts with complete foods, such as yogurt, almonds, and seeds, will help support the health of your liver even more. For instance, a parfait made of Greek yogurt, berries, and chopped nuts is a nutrient-dense, low-glycemic index choice that can satisfy sweet cravings without sacrificing taste. In the end, it all comes down to finding a balance between indulging in sweets and making decisions that support liver health without sacrificing taste.

CHAPTER 7

RICH IN ANTIOXIDANTS MEALS

Bright Fruit And Vegetable Salads

Adding colorful fruit and vegetable salads to your liver-healthy dishes is a fresh and nutrient-dense strategy. The antioxidants included in fruits and vegetables can help the liver, which is essential for detoxification. These vibrantly colored salads offer a range of nutrients that help the body fight off dangerous free radicals. Chlorophyll, a strong antioxidant that helps liver detoxification pathways, is a component of dark, leafy greens like kale and spinach. Furthermore, colorful veggies like tomatoes and bell peppers include vitamins A and C, which boosts the antioxidant content of these salads even more. In addition to adding visual attractiveness to the dish, a varied palette of fruits and vegetables guarantees a wide range of antioxidants, which supports the health of the liver overall.

Berry And Citrus Infused Dishes

When it comes to creating antioxidant-rich, liver-friendly meals, berries, and citrus fruits are particularly potent companions. Anthocyanins and flavonoids, which are abundant in berries and are well-known for their strong antioxidant qualities, include blueberries, strawberries, and raspberries. These substances have been connected to lowering inflammation and oxidative stress, which supports liver health.

Citrus fruits, such as lemons, oranges, and grapefruits, are rich in vitamin C, an essential antioxidant that helps produce glutathione, which is essential for liver detoxification. When these fruits are added to food—whether salads, desserts, or main courses—they not only improve taste but also supply a significant amount of antioxidants that support liver health.

Using Herbs and Spices for Antioxidants:

Using herbs and spices to boost antioxidant levels is a sophisticated and tasty way to create meals that support liver health. Herbs having anti-inflammatory and antioxidant qualities, such as rosemary and turmeric, contain bioactive components. Curcumin, the main ingredient in turmeric, has been researched for its potential to reduce inflammation and liver damage. Similarly, the compound rosmarinic acid found in rosemary has hepatoprotective properties. Adding these herbs to food—such as tea, marinades, or seasonings—not only improves the flavor but also offers a strong antioxidant source. Other important spices are ginger and cinnamon. Ginger has anti-inflammatory qualities, and cinnamon has been associated with increased insulin sensitivity, which indirectly benefits the liver. By carefully combining these herbs and spices, one can make tasty recipes that support liver health by reducing inflammation and oxidative stress.

CHAPTER 8

RECIPES FOR LEAN PROTEIN

Fish- And Poultry-Based Recipes

Including lean protein sources in your diet, such as fish and chicken, can be crucial for supporting liver function. For meals that are good for the liver, poultry like chicken and turkey as well as fatty fish like salmon and mackerel are great options. Essential amino acids, which are the building blocks of proteins required to maintain liver function, are abundant in these proteins.

When cooked without over-frying or the addition of bad fats, poultry offers a lean protein supply that helps maintain muscle mass without overtaxing the liver. Fish, especially those rich in omega-3 fatty acids, has anti-inflammatory properties and may help prevent the buildup of liver fat.

Additionally, these proteins are generally lower in saturated fats, which makes them heart-healthy options. This is important for those with liver problems, which are frequently linked to cardiovascular problems.

Additionally, adding these proteins to meals for liver health might be a delightful experience. Flavored with herbs and spices, baked salmon or grilled chicken not only pleases the palate but also supplies vital nutrients that aid in the liver's detoxifying processes.

Sources Of Plant-Based Protein

There are many protein-rich, plant-based foods that can be tasty and nutritious for individuals looking for liver-healthy recipes.

Chickpeas and lentils are two good plant-based sources of protein. In addition to being high in protein, they are also high in fiber, which supports healthy digestion and aids in blood sugar regulation.

This is an extra advantage for people who have liver problems, which are frequently linked to metabolic problems.

Other plant-based proteins that are easily included in meals that are good for the liver are tofu and tempeh, which are made from soybeans. These choices offer a full spectrum of amino acids and work well in a variety of meals, including salads and stir-fries.

Selecting plant-based proteins instead of animal-based ones will also help you consume less cholesterol and saturated fats, which will ease the burden on your liver and improve your general cardiovascular health.

People can make meals that promote liver function and satisfy a range of tastes and preferences by experimenting with different plant-based protein recipes. This makes eating a liver-friendly diet both approachable and pleasurable.

Managing Protein Consumption For Hepatic Support

For the support of the liver, a balanced protein intake is essential. Although the liver needs proteins for many internal processes, including liver health, an excessive amount might be difficult for the liver to handle. Thus, striking the correct balance is essential.

It's critical to take into account both the amount and type of protein consumed. To keep the liver from being overloaded with more protein than it can effectively digest, portion management is crucial. Additionally, limiting the consumption of harmful lipids that may exacerbate liver inflammation can be achieved by choosing lean protein sources, whether they come from plants or animals.

A balanced approach takes into account the meal's entire composition as well. A well-rounded and nutrient-rich diet is achieved by combining proteins with whole grains, a range of veggies, and healthy fats. This method not only promotes liver function but also gives the body a wide variety of nutrients that are essential for general wellness.

To sum up, the inclusion of plant-based proteins, the prioritization of lean protein sources, and the maintenance of balanced protein consumption are essential elements of liver health recipes.

CHAPITRE 9

LIMITING ADDITIVES AND PROCESSED FOODS

Processed Foods' Effects On Liver Health

Processed foods are quite dangerous for the health of your liver since they are loaded with artificial additives, preservatives, and high amounts of sugar and sodium. A diet high in processed foods can overburden the liver, an essential organ involved in metabolism and detoxification.

An increasing number of processed products include high fructose corn syrup, which has been connected to non-alcoholic fatty liver disease (NAFLD). Overindulgence in refined carbohydrates, which are widely present in processed foods, also adds to the buildup of fat in the liver, which causes inflammation and poor liver function.

Moreover, trans fats, which raise bad cholesterol and cause inflammation, are a common ingredient in processed foods. These bad fats, which are frequently included in baked products, fried foods, and snacks, can cause liver illnesses including cirrhosis. A diet high in whole, unprocessed foods is necessary to promote liver function since the combination of these dangerous ingredients in processed meals produces a perfect storm for liver damage.

Examining Labels And Making Knowledgeable Decisions

Being a careful reader of labels is a crucial first step in supporting liver health. Consumers need to understand food labels since manufacturers frequently use confusing language or cover up dangerous components with other names. Red flags should be raised by high quantities of trans fats, salt, and added sugars.

It's important to choose items with clear ingredient lists, identifiable parts, and little additions.

Furthermore, it's critical to comprehend serving quantities to avoid consuming excessive amounts of dangerous chemicals.

Foods may seem low in fat or sugar per serving, but if portions aren't carefully thought out, the overall effect can be substantial. People can make decisions that are beneficial to their overall health and liver health by making it a practice to read and comprehend food labels.

Handcrafted Alternatives To Processed Favorites

Switching out commercial foods for homemade ones is a good way to support liver function. With this method, people have control over the ingredients and can make sure that only healthy, liver-friendly products are utilized. For example, people can make their snacks with whole grains, nuts, and seeds instead of purchasing store-bought snacks that are heavy in fat and sodium. This improves the snacks' nutritional content while also getting rid of dangerous ingredients.

Likewise, swapping out processed, sugary drinks for homemade, organically flavored ones can drastically cut down on added sugar consumption. A tasty substitute that is refreshing is achieved by adding fruits, herbs, or spices to water. A gourmet mentality and experimenting with homemade versions of processed favorites can help people eat delicious meals and actively maintain the health of their livers. People are now more empowered to take charge of their diets and make decisions that support the health of their livers because of the shift towards whole, nutrient-dense meals.

CHAPTER 10

LIVER FUNCTION IN PARTICULAR DIETS

<u>Vegetarian Recipes That Are Liver-Friendly</u>

For general health, liver health maintenance is essential, and vegetarians can find a variety of liver-friendly recipes to help them achieve this. Plant-based diets high in fiber, antioxidants, and other nutrients are frequently the focus of vegetarian options. Beetroot is one such component, well-known for its ability to cleanse the liver. Beetroot added to salads or smoothies can help support the liver's detoxifying activities.

Incorporating cruciferous vegetables, such as Brussels sprouts and broccoli, also supplies sulfur compounds that aid in the pathways involved in liver detoxification. These veggies make a delicious and wholesome side dish when roasted with olive oil and seasoning, which is a great recipe.

Chickpeas and lentils are two legumes that are great providers of fiber and protein. They can be added to salads, stews, and soups to make filling, liver-friendly dishes.

Liver function is significantly impacted by healthy fats. For example, avocados are a good source of monounsaturated fats and can be sliced into whole-grain bread or mashed into guacamole. Omega-3 fatty acids from nuts and seeds, particularly flaxseeds and walnuts, are good for the liver. Think about adding these to homemade energy bars, cereal, or smoothies.

In summary, a wide variety of plant-based foods, such as beetroots, cruciferous vegetables, legumes, avocados, nuts, and seeds, are featured in vegetarian dishes that are liver-friendly. Within the parameters of a vegetarian diet, people can make tasty meals that promote liver health by embracing these items.

Recipes Designed With Dietary Constraints In Mind

Following recipes that are good for the liver gets more complicated when you take people with special dietary needs into account. Finding safe substitutes that support liver function is essential for people with dietary restrictions like gluten sensitivity or intolerance.

Gluten-free quinoa can be used as a flexible salad or bowl basis. Because of its high protein content, it's a filling and healthy choice. Furthermore, those who are intolerant to lactose can use dairy-free substitutes in recipes, such as almond or coconut milk, without sacrificing taste or nutrients.

In low-sodium diets, which are frequently advised for liver health, herbs and spices play a crucial role in enhancing flavor. Fresh herbs such as cilantro, parsley, or dill can be used to season food, giving it a flavor boost without using too much salt.

Recipes that address both illnesses are beneficial for those with diabetes, another prevalent health issue that is frequently associated with liver function. Think about preparing meals with lots of non-starchy veggies, nutritious grains, and lean proteins. An array of vibrant vegetables and quinoa combined with grilled fish or tofu create a healthy and liver-friendly lunch.

Essentially, recipes designed for people with dietary limitations give preference to substitutions that meet particular requirements, such as low-sodium seasoning, dairy-free options, gluten-free grains, and options that are blood sugar-friendly for people with diabetes.

Modifying Customary Recipes to Promote Liver Health

Making classic meals into variants that promote liver function is the process of adapting traditional foods for liver health. The substitution of lean proteins for fatty meats is one such alteration. For instance, replacing lean ground beef in a chili recipe with lean ground turkey preserves the dish's heartiness while lowering the amount of saturated fat.

Whole grains have a higher fiber level that promotes digestive health and helps with toxin removal, so they can be used in place of refined grains in classic recipes. You can substitute brown rice or quinoa for white rice to up the nutritional content and give the dish a nuttier taste.

Cutting back on added sugars is another important change. Traditional recipes frequently have high sugar content, which can lead to the buildup of liver fat. This problem is lessened by choosing unsweetened substitutes or using natural sweeteners like honey or maple syrup sparingly.

Furthermore, adding more vegetables to classic dishes improves their profile of liver-friendliness. Vitamins and minerals are added when, for example, extra vegetables are added to pasta recipes or a range of colorful vegetables are added to stir-fries.

To sum up, modifying classic recipes to promote liver health entails making thoughtful replacements, such as selecting lean proteins, adding whole grains, cutting back on added sweets, and adding more vegetables. These changes convert well-known dishes into liver-friendly choices, which improves health in general.

CHAPTER 11

ORGANIZING YOUR MEALS FOR LIVER HEALTH

<u>Weekly Meal Plans For Supporting The Liver</u>

A key component of maintaining liver health is creating a weekly diet plan that is specific to liver wellness. Dietary decisions are essential to the liver's health because it is responsible for cleansing the body and metabolizing nutrients. Nutrient-rich foods that support liver function and general health should be the main focus of any weekly meal plan for liver maintenance.

It's important to include a range of vibrant vegetables since they offer vital minerals and antioxidants. Carrots, broccoli, and other cruciferous vegetables, as well as dark leafy greens, help the liver detoxify.

Furthermore, adding fruits like citrus and berries that are rich in antioxidants might help strengthen the liver's defenses against dangerous toxins.

Protein sources should be carefully selected to reduce hepatic stress. Important amino acids can be obtained without consuming too much-saturated fat from plant-based foods like beans and legumes or lean meats like skinless chicken and fish. Sufficient hydration is also essential because it helps the liver eliminate toxins.

Moreover, a sizable component of the weekly food plan should consist of healthy grains and complex carbs. Choosing foods such as brown rice, quinoa, and whole wheat bread releases energy gradually, reducing blood sugar fluctuations and maintaining a steady metabolic environment for the liver.

Advice For Preparing And Batch Cooking

Maintaining a diet that is healthy to the liver requires effective meal preparation, and batch cooking is a useful tactic in this regard. By preparing greater quantities of meals ahead of time, batch cooking helps to promote consistency in dietary choices while also saving time. This strategy can simplify the addition of vital nutrients for those concerned with liver health while lowering the possibility of choosing less healthful options when convenience calls for it.

Prioritizing recipes that use liver-supporting components is crucial when batch cooking for liver well-being. Pick dishes that include nutritious grains, lots of veggies, and lean proteins. Soups, stews, and stir-fries are examples of batch-cooking mainstays that allow for a wide variety of ingredients and flavors to be added while still maintaining a healthy dinner.

To maintain the nutritional value of the cooked meals, effective batch cooking also requires adequate storage. Invest in high-quality storage containers to minimize the need for preservatives and keep food fresh.

An orderly rotation system can be maintained by labeling and dating the containers, guaranteeing that the older batches are finished first.

Making Nutrient-Dense, Balanced Meals

A key element of liver fitness is maintaining a nutrient-dense composition of each meal and balancing macronutrients. An adequate ratio of proteins, carbs, and fats is included in a balanced diet to maintain general health and provide long-lasting energy.

Because they aid in tissue regeneration and the synthesis of enzymes, proteins are necessary for liver function. A well-rounded consumption of amino acids is ensured by incorporating a range of protein sources, including lean meats, fish, eggs, and plant-based alternatives. Pay attention to portion proportions to spare your liver from needless strain.

Stable blood sugar levels are mostly dependent on carbs, particularly complex carbohydrates. Excellent sources of complex carbohydrates that also provide fiber and vital nutrients to support digestive health are whole grains, legumes, and vegetables.

For optimal nutrient absorption and general health, include healthy fats such as those in nuts, avocados, and olive oil. Additionally, these fats aid in satiety, which helps people avoid overindulging in less healthful foods.

To increase the amount of vitamins, minerals, and antioxidants in nutrient-dense meals, concentrate on including a range of vibrant fruits and vegetables. Adding different herbs and spices to food not only improves flavor but also has other health advantages.

Through the regular preparation of well-balanced and nutrient-dense meals, people can take an active role in maintaining the health of their livers while also having a varied and fulfilling gastronomic experience.

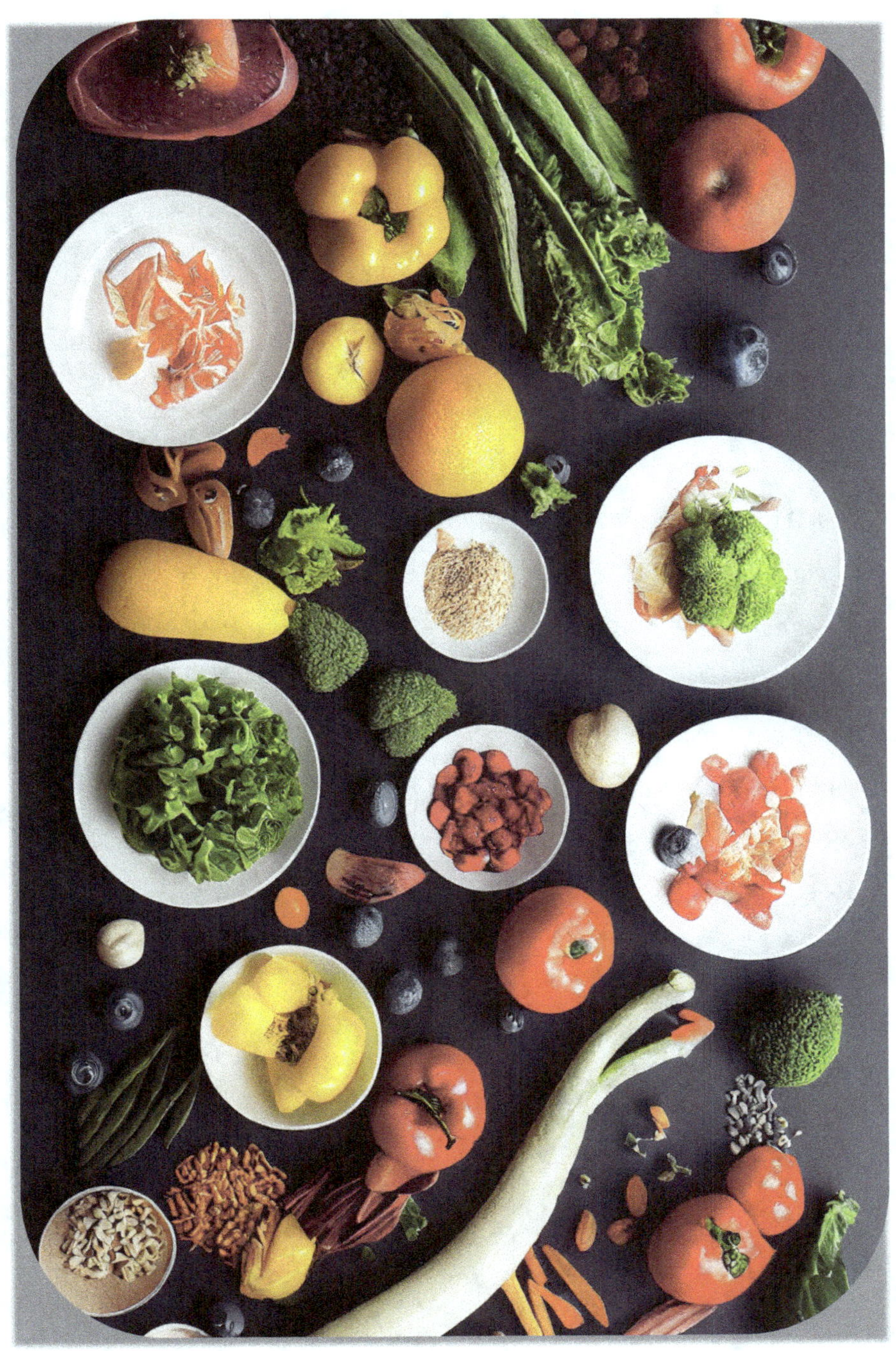

CHAPTER 12

28 DAY MEAL PLAN

Day 1

Breakfast: Spinach And Mushroom Omelette

Servings: 1

Prep Time: 10 minutes

Ingredients:

- *3 eggs*

- 1 cup spinach, chopped

- 1/2 cup mushrooms, sliced

- 1/4 cup onion, diced

- Salt and pepper to taste

- 1 teaspoon olive oil

Cooking Instructions:

1. In a bowl, whisk the eggs with salt and pepper.

2. Heat olive oil in a non-stick skillet over medium heat.

3. Add the onions and mushrooms to the skillet and sauté until softened.

4. Add the chopped spinach and cook until wilted.

5. Pour the whisked eggs over the vegetables in the skillet.

6. Cook until the eggs are set, then fold the omelette in half and serve hot.

Lunch: Turkey And Vegetable Stir-Fry

Servings: 2

Prep Time: 15 minutes

Ingredients:

- 1/2 lb turkey breast, thinly sliced

- 2 cups mixed vegetables (such as bell peppers, broccoli, carrots)

- 2 cloves garlic, minced

- 2 tablespoons low-sodium soy sauce

- 1 tablespoon olive oil

- Salt and pepper to taste

Cooking Instructions:

1. Heat olive oil in a wok or large skillet over high heat.

2. Add the minced garlic and cook until fragrant.

3. Add the sliced turkey breast and stir-fry until cooked through.

4. Add the mixed vegetables to the skillet and continue stir-frying until tender-crisp.

5. Stir in the soy sauce, salt, and pepper, and cook for another minute.

6. Serve hot.

Dinner: Baked Cod with Asparagus

Servings: 2

prep time: 10 minutes

Ingredients:

- 2 cod fillets

- 1 bunch asparagus, trimmed

- 2 tablespoons lemon juice

- 2 cloves garlic, minced

- 1 tablespoon olive oil

- Salt and pepper to taste

- Servings: 2

Cooking Instructions:

1. Preheat the oven to 400°F (200°C).

2. Place the cod fillets and asparagus on a baking sheet.

3. In a small bowl, mix together lemon juice, minced garlic, olive oil, salt, and pepper.

4. Drizzle the lemon-garlic mixture over the cod fillets and asparagus.

5. Bake in the preheated oven for 12-15 minutes, or until the fish flakes easily with a fork.

6. Serve hot.

Snack: Almonds And Apple Slices

Servings: 1

- 1/4 cup almonds

- 1 medium apple, sliced

Prep Time: 2 minutes

Ingredients:

Cooking Instructions:

Day 2

Breakfast: Berry Smoothie Bowl

Servings: 1

Prep Time: 5 minutes

Ingredients:

 - 1 cup mixed berries (such as strawberries, blueberries, raspberries)

 - 1 frozen banana

 - 1/2 cup spinach

 - 1/2 cup unsweetened almond milk

 - 1 tablespoon chia seeds

Toppings: sliced banana, granola, shredded coconut

Cooking Instructions:

1. In a blender, combine mixed berries, frozen banana, spinach, almond milk, and chia seeds.

2. Blend until smooth and creamy.

3. Pour the smoothie into a bowl and top with sliced banana, granola, and shredded coconut.

1. Enjoy a handful of almonds with apple slices for a satisfying snack

Lunch: Lentil and Vegetable Soup

Servings: 4

Prep Time: 10 minutes

Ingredients:

 - 1 cup dried lentils, rinsed

 - 4 cups vegetable broth

 - 1 onion, diced

 - 2 carrots, diced

 - 2 celery stalks, diced

 - 2 cloves garlic, minced

 - 1 teaspoon cumin

 - 1 teaspoon paprika

 - Salt and pepper to taste

Cooking Instructions:

1. In a large pot, combine lentils, vegetable broth, diced onion,

carrots, celery, minced garlic, cumin, paprika, salt, and pepper.

2. Bring the soup to a boil, then reduce the heat to low and simmer for 20-25 minutes, or until the lentils and vegetables are tender.

3. Adjust seasoning if needed.

4. Serve hot.

Dinner: Grilled Chicken with Roasted Vegetables

Servings: 2

Prep Time: 15 minutes

Ingredients:

- 2 boneless, skinless chicken breasts

- 2 cups mixed vegetables (such as bell peppers, zucchini, cherry tomatoes)

- 2 tablespoons olive oil

- 2 cloves garlic, minced

- 1 teaspoon Italian seasoning

- Salt and pepper to taste

Cooking Instructions:

1. Preheat the grill or grill pan over medium-high heat.

2. Season the chicken breasts with olive oil, minced garlic, Italian seasoning, salt, and pepper.

3. Grill the chicken for 6-7 minutes per side, or until cooked through.

4. In a separate bowl, toss the mixed vegetables with olive oil, salt, and pepper.

5. Spread the vegetables on a baking sheet and roast in the oven at 400°F (200°C) for 15-20 minutes, or until tender.

6. Serve the grilled chicken with roasted vegetables.

Snack: Cottage Cheese with Pineapple

Servings: 1

Prep Time: 2 minutes

Ingredients:

- 1/2 cup low-fat cottage cheese

- 1/2 cup fresh pineapple chunks

Cooking Instructions:

1. Enjoy cottage cheese topped with fresh pineapple chunks for a nutritious snack.

Day 3

Breakfast: Veggie Egg Muffins

Servings: 3 (2 muffins per serving)

Prep Time: 10 minutes

Ingredients:

- 6 eggs

- 1/2 cup spinach, chopped

- 1/4 cup bell peppers, diced

- 1/4 cup onion, diced

- 1/4 cup cherry tomatoes, halved

- Salt and pepper to taste

Cooking Instructions:

1. Preheat the oven to 350°F (175°C) and grease a muffin tin.

2. In a bowl, whisk together eggs, chopped spinach, diced bell peppers, diced onion, cherry tomatoes, salt, and pepper.

3. Pour the egg mixture evenly into the muffin tin.

4. Bake for 20-25 minutes, or until the egg muffins are set and lightly golden.

5. Allow them to cool slightly before removing from the muffin tin. Serve warm.

Lunch: Quinoa Salad with Chickpeas

Servings: 2

Prep Time: 15 minutes

Ingredients:

- 1 cup quinoa, cooked

- 1 can chickpeas, rinsed and drained

- 1 cucumber, diced

- 1/2 cup cherry tomatoes, halved

- 1/4 cup red onion, finely chopped

- 2 tablespoons fresh parsley, chopped

- Juice of 1 lemon

- 2 tablespoons olive oil

- Salt and pepper to taste

Cooking Instructions:

1. In a large bowl, combine cooked quinoa, chickpeas, diced cucumber, cherry tomatoes, chopped red onion, and chopped parsley.

2. In a small bowl, whisk together lemon juice, olive oil, salt, and pepper to make the dressing.`

3. Pour the dressing over the quinoa salad and toss to coat evenly.

4. Serve chilled or at room temperature.

Dinner: Turkey Meatballs with Zucchini Noodles

Servings: 2

Prep Time: 20 minutes

Ingredients:

- 1/2 lb ground turkey

- 1/4 cup breadcrumbs

- 1 egg

- 2 cloves garlic, minced

- 1/4 cup grated Parmesan cheese

- 1 tablespoon fresh parsley, chopped

- Salt and pepper to taste

- 2 medium zucchinis

- Olive oil

- Marinara sauce (optional)

Cooking Instructions:

1. In a bowl, combine ground turkey, breadcrumbs, egg, minced garlic, grated Parmesan cheese, chopped parsley, salt, and pepper. Mix until well combined.

2. Shape the turkey mixture into meatballs.

3. Heat olive oil in a skillet over medium heat. Add the meatballs and cook until browned on all sides and cooked through.

4. While the meatballs are cooking, spiralize the zucchinis to make noodles.

5. In a separate skillet, heat olive oil over medium heat. Add the zucchini noodles and cook for 2-3 minutes, or until tender.

6. Serve the turkey meatballs over the zucchini noodles with marinara sauce if desired.

Snack: Whole Grain Crackers with Hummus

Servings: 1

Prep Time: 2 minutes

Ingredients:

- Whole grain crackers

- Hummus

Cooking Instructions:

1. Enjoy whole grain crackers with hummus for a satisfying snack.

Day 4

Breakfast: Greek Yogurt Parfait

Servings: 1

Prep Time: 5 minutes

Ingredients:

- 1 cup Greek yogurt

- 1/2 cup granola

- 1/2 cup mixed berries (such as strawberries, blueberries, raspberries)

- 1 tablespoon honey (optional)

Cooking Instructions:

1. In a glass or bowl, layer Greek yogurt, granola, and mixed berries.

2. Drizzle with honey if desired.

3. Repeat layering if desired.

4. Serve immediately.

Lunch: Spinach and Chickpea Salad

- Servings: 2

- Prep Time: 10 minutes

Ingredients:

- 2 cups baby spinach

- 1/2 cup cherry tomatoes, halved

- 1/2 cup cucumber, diced

- 1/4 cup red onion, thinly sliced

- 1/2 cup canned chickpeas, rinsed and drained

- 2 tablespoons feta cheese, crumbled

- 2 tablespoons balsamic vinaigrette

Cooking Instructions:

1. In a large bowl, combine baby spinach, cherry tomatoes, diced cucumber, sliced red onion, and chickpeas.

2. Drizzle with balsamic vinaigrette and toss to coat evenly.

3. Top with crumbled feta cheese before serving.

Dinner: Baked Salmon with Steamed Broccoli

Servings: 2

Prep Time: 10 minutes

- Ingredients:

  - 2 salmon fillets

  - 1 tablespoon olive oil

  - 1 teaspoon lemon zest

  - 1 teaspoon dried dill

  - Salt and pepper to taste

  - 2 cups broccoli florets

- **Cooking Instructions:**

1. Preheat the oven to 375°F (190°C).

2. Place the salmon fillets on a baking sheet lined with parchment paper.

3. In a small bowl, mix together olive oil, lemon zest, dried dill, salt, and pepper.

4. Brush the olive oil mixture over the salmon fillets.

5. Bake in the preheated oven for 12-15 minutes, or until the salmon is cooked through and flakes easily with a fork.

6. While the salmon is baking, steam the broccoli until tender-crisp.

7. Serve the baked salmon with steamed broccoli on the side.

Snack: Carrot Sticks with Hummus

Servings: 1

Prep Time: 2 minutes

Ingredients:

  - Carrot sticks

  - Hummus

Cooking Instructions:

1. Enjoy carrot sticks with hummus for a crunchy and satisfying snack.

Day 5

Breakfast: Banana Walnut Oatmeal

Servings: 1

Prep Time: 5 minutes

Ingredients:

- 1/2 cup rolled oats

- 1 cup water or milk of choice

- 1 ripe banana, mashed

- 2 tablespoons chopped walnuts

- 1 tablespoon honey or maple syrup (optional)

Cooking Instructions:

1. In a saucepan, bring water or milk to a boil.

2. Stir in rolled oats and reduce heat to simmer.

3. Cook for 5 minutes, stirring occasionally, until oats are creamy and tender.

4. Stir in mashed banana and chopped walnuts.

5. Sweeten with honey or maple syrup if desired.

6. Serve hot.

Lunch: Turkey and Avocado Wrap

Servings: 2

Prep Time: 10 minutes

Ingredients:

- 2 large whole grain wraps or tortillas

- 1/2 lb sliced turkey breast

- 1 ripe avocado, sliced

- 1 cup mixed salad greens

- 1/4 cup shredded carrots

- 2 tablespoons Greek yogurt or mayo (optional)

Cooking Instructions:

1. Lay out the wraps or tortillas on a flat surface.

2. Layer sliced turkey breast, avocado slices, mixed salad greens, and shredded carrots on each wrap.

3. Drizzle with Greek yogurt or mayo if using.

4. Roll up the wraps tightly and cut in half diagonally.

5. Serve immediately or wrap in foil for later.

Dinner: Vegetable Stir-Fry with Tofu

Servings: 2

Prep Time: 15 minutes

Ingredients:

- 1 block firm tofu, pressed and cubed

- 2 cups mixed vegetables (such as bell peppers, broccoli, snap peas, carrots)

- 2 cloves garlic, minced

- 2 tablespoons low-sodium soy sauce

- 1 tablespoon hoisin sauce

- 1 tablespoon sesame oil

- Cooked brown rice or quinoa for serving

Cooking Instructions:

1. Heat sesame oil in a large skillet or wok over medium-high heat.

2. Add minced garlic and cubed tofu to the skillet. Cook until tofu is golden brown on all sides.

3. Add mixed vegetables to the skillet and stir-fry until they are tender-crisp.

4. In a small bowl, mix together low-sodium soy sauce and hoisin sauce. Pour over the tofu and vegetables.

5. Cook for another 2-3 minutes, stirring constantly, until everything is coated in the sauce.

6. Serve vegetable stir-fry over cooked brown rice or quinoa.

Snack: Cottage Cheese with Sliced Peaches

Servings: 1

Prep Time: 2 minutes

Ingredients:

- 1/2 cup low-fat cottage cheese

- 1 ripe peach, sliced

Cooking Instructions:

1. Enjoy cottage cheese topped with sliced peaches for a refreshing snack.

Day 6

Breakfast: Veggie Scramble

Servings: 1

Prep Time: 10 minutes

Ingredients:

- 2 eggs

- 1/4 cup diced bell peppers

- 1/4 cup diced tomatoes

- 1/4 cup diced onions

- 1/4 cup chopped spinach

- Salt and pepper to taste

Cooking Instructions:

1. Heat a non-stick skillet over medium heat.

2. Add diced onions and bell peppers to the skillet and sauté until softened.

3. Add diced tomatoes and chopped spinach to the skillet and cook until spinach is wilted.

4. In a bowl, beat eggs with salt and pepper.

5. Pour the beaten eggs into the skillet with the vegetables.

6. Cook, stirring occasionally, until the eggs are scrambled and cooked to your liking.

7. Serve hot.

Lunch: Quinoa and Black Bean Salad

Servings: 2

Prep Time: 15 minutes

Ingredients:

- 1 cup quinoa, cooked

- 1 can black beans, rinsed and drained

- 1 red bell pepper, diced

- 1/4 cup red onion, finely chopped

- 1/4 cup cilantro, chopped

- Juice of 1 lime

- 2 tablespoons olive oil

- Salt and pepper to taste

Cooking Instructions:

1. In a large bowl, combine cooked quinoa, black beans, diced red bell pepper, chopped red onion, and chopped cilantro.

2. In a small bowl, whisk together lime juice, olive oil, salt, and pepper to make the dressing.

3. Pour the dressing over the quinoa salad and toss to coat evenly.

4. Serve chilled or at room temperature.

Dinner: **Baked Chicken with Sweet Potato Mash**

Servings: 2

Prep Time: 15 minutes

Ingredients:

- 2 boneless, skinless chicken breasts

- 2 medium sweet potatoes, peeled and cubed

- 2 tablespoons olive oil

- 2 cloves garlic, minced

- 1 teaspoon paprika

- Salt and pepper to taste

Cooking Instructions:

1. Preheat the oven to 400°F (200°C).

2. Place the chicken breasts on a baking sheet lined with parchment paper.

3. In a small bowl, mix together olive oil, minced garlic, paprika, salt, and pepper.

4. Brush the olive oil mixture over the chicken breasts.

5. Bake in the preheated oven for 20-25 minutes, or until the chicken is cooked through and no longer pink in the center.

6. While the chicken is baking, boil the sweet potato cubes in a pot of water until tender.

7. Drain the sweet potatoes and mash them with a fork or potato masher until smooth.

8. Season the sweet potato mash with salt and pepper to taste.

9. Serve the baked chicken with sweet potato mash on the side.

Snack: **Whole Grain Crackers with Guacamole**

- **Servings: 1**

- **Prep Time: 2 minutes**

- **Ingredients:**

- Whole grain crackers

- Guacamole

1. Enjoy whole grain crackers with guacamole for a satisfying snack.

Day 7

Breakfast: Berry Chia Seed Pudding

Ingredients:

- 1/4 cup chia seeds

- 1 cup unsweetened almond milk (or any milk of choice)

- 1/2 teaspoon vanilla extract

- 1 tablespoon honey or maple syrup (optional)

- 1/2 cup mixed berries (such as strawberries, blueberries, raspberries)

Servings: 1

Prep Time: 5 minutes (plus chilling time)

Cooking Instructions:

1. In a bowl, mix chia seeds, almond milk, vanilla extract, and honey (if using).

2. Stir well to combine and let sit for 5 minutes.

3. Stir again to break up any clumps of chia seeds.

4. Cover the bowl and refrigerate for at least 2 hours or overnight, until the mixture thickens and resembles pudding.

5. Before serving, top the chia seed pudding with mixed berries.

Lunch: Turkey and Vegetable Wrap

Ingredients:

- 2 large whole grain wraps or tortillas

- 1/2 lb sliced turkey breast

- 1/2 cup hummus

- 1 cup mixed salad greens

- 1/4 cup shredded carrots

- 1/4 cup cucumber, sliced

1. Lay out the wraps or tortillas on a flat surface.

2. Spread hummus evenly over each wrap.

3. Layer sliced turkey breast, mixed salad greens, shredded carrots, and sliced cucumber on each wrap.

4. Roll up the wraps tightly and cut in half diagonally.

5. Serve immediately or wrap in foil for later.

Dinner: Grilled Shrimp with Quinoa Salad

Ingredients:

- 1/2 lb large shrimp, peeled and deveined

- 1 tablespoon olive oil

- 1 teaspoon smoked paprika

- 1/2 teaspoon garlic powder

- Salt and pepper to taste

- 1 cup quinoa, cooked

- 1/2 cup cherry tomatoes, halved

- 1/4 cup cucumber, diced

- 1/4 cup red onion, finely chopped

- 2 tablespoons fresh parsley, chopped

- Juice of 1 lemon

- 2 tablespoons olive oil

Servings: 2

Prep Time: 15 minutes

Cooking Instructions:

1. Preheat the grill or grill pan over medium-high heat.

2. In a bowl, toss shrimp with olive oil, smoked paprika, garlic powder, salt, and pepper.

3. Thread shrimp onto skewers.

4. Grill shrimp for 2-3 minutes per side, or until pink and cooked through.

5. In a large bowl, combine cooked quinoa, cherry tomatoes, diced cucumber, chopped red onion, and chopped parsley.

6. In a small bowl, whisk together lemon juice and olive oil to make the dressing.

7. Pour the dressing over the quinoa salad and toss to coat evenly.

8. Serve grilled shrimp over quinoa salad.

Snack: Apple Slices with Almond Butter

Ingredients:

- 1 apple, sliced

- 2 tablespoons almond butter

Servings: 1

Prep Time: 2 minutes

Cooking Instructions:

1. Enjoy apple slices with almond butter for a satisfying snack.

Day 8

Breakfast: Spinach and Feta Egg Muffins

Ingredients:

- 6 eggs

- 1 cup baby spinach, chopped

- 1/4 cup crumbled feta cheese

- Salt and pepper to taste

Servings: 3 (2 muffins per serving)

Prep Time: 10 minutes

Cooking Instructions:

1. Preheat the oven to 350°F (175°C) and grease a muffin tin.

2. In a bowl, whisk together eggs, chopped baby spinach, crumbled feta cheese, salt, and pepper.

3. Pour the egg mixture evenly into the muffin tin.

4. Bake for 20-25 minutes, or until the egg muffins are set and lightly golden.

5. Allow them to cool slightly before removing from the muffin tin. Serve warm.

Lunch: Mediterranean Chickpea Salad

Ingredients:

- 1 can chickpeas, rinsed and drained

- 1 cucumber, diced

- 1 cup cherry tomatoes, halved

- 1/4 cup red onion, finely chopped

- 1/4 cup Kalamata olives, pitted and sliced

- 2 tablespoons fresh parsley, chopped

- Juice of 1 lemon

- 2 tablespoons olive oil

- Salt and pepper to taste

Servings: 2

Prep Time: 10 minutes

Cooking Instructions:

1. In a large bowl, combine chickpeas, diced cucumber, cherry tomatoes, chopped red onion, sliced Kalamata olives, and chopped parsley.

2. In a small bowl, whisk together lemon juice, olive oil, salt, and pepper to make the dressing.

3. Pour the dressing over the chickpea salad and toss to coat evenly.

4. Serve chilled or at room temperature.

Dinner: Baked Cod with Mediterranean Vegetables

Ingredients:

- 2 cod fillets

- 1 cup cherry tomatoes, halved

- 1/2 cup Kalamata olives, pitted

- 1/4 cup red onion, thinly sliced

- 2 cloves garlic, minced

- 2 tablespoons olive oil

- 1 tablespoon balsamic vinegar

- Salt and pepper to taste

Servings: 2

Prep Time: 15 minutes

Cooking Instructions:

1. Preheat the oven to 400°F (200°C).

2. In a baking dish, combine cherry tomatoes, Kalamata olives, thinly sliced red onion, minced garlic, olive oil, balsamic vinegar, salt, and pepper.

3. Toss everything together to coat evenly.

4. Place the cod fillets on top of the vegetable mixture.

5. Drizzle olive oil over the cod fillets and season with salt and pepper.

6. Bake in the preheated oven for 15-20 minutes, or until the fish flakes easily with a fork and the vegetables are tender.

7. Serve hot.

Snack: Greek Yogurt with Mixed Nuts

- Ingredients:

- 1 cup Greek yogurt

- 1/4 cup mixed nuts (such as almonds, walnuts, cashews)

Servings: 1

Prep Time: 2 minutes

Cooking Instructions:

1. Enjoy Greek yogurt topped with mixed nuts for a protein-rich snack.

Day 9

Breakfast: Banana Almond Smoothie

Ingredients:

- 1 ripe banana

- 1 cup almond milk

- 2 tablespoons almond butter

- 1 tablespoon honey or maple syrup (optional)

- Ice cubes (optional)

Servings: 1

Prep Time: 5 minutes

Cooking Instructions:

1. In a blender, combine ripe banana, almond milk, almond butter, and honey or maple syrup if using.

2. Add ice cubes if desired for a colder smoothie.

3. Blend until smooth and creamy.

4. Pour into a glass and enjoy immediately.

Lunch: Caprese Salad

Ingredients:

- 2 large tomatoes, sliced

- 1 ball fresh mozzarella cheese, sliced

- Fresh basil leaves

- 2 tablespoons balsamic glaze

- Salt and pepper to taste

Servings: 2

Prep Time: 5 minutes

Cooking Instructions:

1. Arrange tomato slices and mozzarella slices alternately on a plate.

2. Tuck fresh basil leaves between the tomato and mozzarella slices.

3. Drizzle balsamic glaze over the salad.

4. Season with salt and pepper to taste.

5. Serve immediately as a refreshing salad.

Dinner: Lemon Herb Grilled Chicken

Ingredients:

- 2 boneless, skinless chicken breasts

- 2 tablespoons olive oil

- 2 cloves garlic, minced

- Zest and juice of 1 lemon

- 1 tablespoon fresh herbs (such as rosemary, thyme, or parsley), chopped

- Salt and pepper to taste

Servings: 2

Prep Time: 10 minutes

Cooking Instructions:

1. In a small bowl, whisk together olive oil, minced garlic, lemon zest, lemon juice, chopped fresh herbs, salt, and pepper.

2. Place chicken breasts in a shallow dish and pour the marinade over them, turning to coat evenly.

3. Cover and refrigerate for at least 30 minutes, or up to 4 hours.

4. Preheat the grill to medium-high heat.

5. Remove chicken from marinade and discard excess marinade.

6. Grill chicken for 6-8 minutes per side, or until cooked through and no longer pink in the center.

7. Serve hot with your choice of side dishes.

Snack: Veggie Sticks with Hummus

Ingredients:

- Carrot sticks

- Celery sticks

- Cucumber sticks

- Hummus

Servings: 1

Prep Time: 5 minutes

Cooking Instructions:

1. Arrange carrot sticks, celery sticks, and cucumber sticks on a plate.

2. Serve with hummus for dipping.

3. Enjoy this crunchy and nutritious snack.

Day 10

Breakfast: Blueberry Almond Overnight Oats

Ingredients:

- 1/2 cup rolled oats

- 1/2 cup almond milk

- 1/4 cup Greek yogurt

- 1/4 cup fresh blueberries

- 1 tablespoon almond butter

- 1 teaspoon honey or maple syrup (optional)

Servings: 1

Prep Time: 5 minutes (plus overnight soaking)

Cooking Instructions:

1. In a jar or container, combine rolled oats, almond milk, Greek yogurt, almond butter, and honey or maple syrup if using.

2. Stir well to combine all ingredients.

3. Gently fold in fresh blueberries.

4. Cover and refrigerate overnight.

5. In the morning, give the oats a stir and enjoy cold or warmed up.

Lunch: Turkey and Avocado Salad

Ingredients:

- 4 oz sliced turkey breast

- 1/2 avocado, sliced

- 2 cups mixed salad greens

- 1/4 cup cherry tomatoes, halved

- 1/4 cup cucumber, sliced

- 2 tablespoons balsamic vinaigrette

Servings: 1

Prep Time: 10 minutes

Cooking Instructions:

1. Arrange mixed salad greens on a plate.

2. Top with sliced turkey breast, avocado slices, cherry tomatoes, and cucumber slices.

3. Drizzle balsamic vinaigrette over the salad.

4. Toss gently to combine, and serve immediately.

Dinner: Veggie Stir-Fry with Tofu

Ingredients:

- 1 block firm tofu, pressed and cubed

- 2 cups mixed vegetables (such as bell peppers, broccoli, snap peas, carrots)

- 2 cloves garlic, minced

- 2 tablespoons low-sodium soy sauce

- 1 tablespoon hoisin sauce

- 1 tablespoon sesame oil

- Cooked brown rice for serving

Servings: 2

Prep Time: 15 minutes

Cooking Instructions:

1. Heat sesame oil in a large skillet or wok over medium-high heat.

2. Add minced garlic and cubed tofu to the skillet. Cook until tofu is golden brown on all sides.

3. Add mixed vegetables to the skillet and stir-fry until they are tender-crisp.

4. In a small bowl, mix together low-sodium soy sauce and hoisin sauce. Pour over the tofu and vegetables.

5. Cook for another 2-3 minutes, stirring constantly, until everything is coated in the sauce.

6. Serve vegetable stir-fry over cooked brown rice.

Snack: Greek Yogurt with Berries

Ingredients:

- 1/2 cup Greek yogurt

- 1/4 cup mixed berries (such as strawberries, blueberries, raspberries)

Servings: 1

Prep Time: 2 minutes

Cooking Instructions:

1. Enjoy Greek yogurt topped with mixed berries for a quick and nutritious snack.

Day 11

Breakfast: Spinach and Mushroom Omelette

Ingredients:

- 2 eggs

- 1/4 cup sliced mushrooms

- 1/4 cup baby spinach leaves

- 2 tablespoons shredded cheese (such as cheddar or feta)

- Salt and pepper to taste

- Cooking spray or olive oil

Servings: 1

Prep Time: 5 minutes

Cooking Instructions:

1. In a bowl, beat the eggs and season with salt and pepper.

2. Heat a non-stick skillet over medium heat and lightly coat with cooking spray or olive oil.

3. Add sliced mushrooms to the skillet and sauté until golden brown.

4. Add baby spinach leaves to the skillet and cook until wilted.

5. Pour the beaten eggs over the mushrooms and spinach.

6. Cook until the edges start to set, then gently lift the edges with a spatula and tilt the skillet to let the uncooked eggs flow to the bottom.

7. Sprinkle shredded cheese over one half of the omelette.

8. Fold the other half of the omelette over the cheese.

9. Cook for another minute or until the cheese is melted and the omelette is cooked through.

10. Slide the omelette onto a plate and serve hot.

Lunch: Quinoa and Black Bean Stuffed Bell Peppers

Ingredients:

- 2 large bell peppers, halved and seeds removed

- 1 cup cooked quinoa

- 1 can black beans, rinsed and drained

- 1/2 cup corn kernels (fresh or frozen)

- 1/4 cup diced tomatoes

- 1/4 cup diced red onion

- 1 teaspoon cumin

- 1/2 teaspoon chili powder

- Salt and pepper to taste

- Optional toppings: shredded cheese, avocado, salsa, Greek yogurt

Servings: 2

Prep Time: 15 minutes

Cooking Instructions:

1. Preheat the oven to 375°F (190°C).

2. In a large bowl, mix together cooked quinoa, black beans, corn kernels, diced tomatoes, diced red onion, cumin, chili powder, salt, and pepper.

3. Stuff each bell pepper half with the quinoa and black bean mixture.

4. Place stuffed bell peppers in a baking dish.

5. Cover the dish with aluminum foil and bake for 25-30 minutes, or until the bell peppers are tender.

6. Remove the foil and sprinkle shredded cheese over the stuffed bell peppers, if desired.

7. Bake for an additional 5 minutes, or until the cheese is melted and bubbly.

8. Serve hot with optional toppings like avocado, salsa, or Greek yogurt.

Dinner: Lemon Garlic Shrimp Pasta

Ingredients:

- 8 oz whole wheat spaghetti or pasta of choice

- 1/2 lb large shrimp, peeled and deveined

- 2 tablespoons olive oil

- 3 cloves garlic, minced

- Zest and juice of 1 lemon

- 1/4 cup chopped fresh parsley

- Salt and pepper to taste

Servings: 2

Prep Time: 15 minutes

Cooking Instructions:

1. Cook pasta according to package instructions until al dente. Drain and set aside.

2. In a large skillet, heat olive oil over medium heat.

3. Add minced garlic to the skillet and sauté for 1 minute, or until fragrant.

4. Add shrimp to the skillet and cook for 2-3 minutes on each side, or until pink and cooked through.

5. Stir in lemon zest and lemon juice.

6. Add cooked pasta to the skillet and toss to coat evenly.

7. Season with salt and pepper to taste.

8. Sprinkle chopped fresh parsley over the pasta and shrimp before serving.

9. Serve hot.

Snack: Celery Sticks with Peanut Butter

Ingredients:

- Celery sticks

- Peanut butter

Servings: 1

Prep Time: 2 minutes

Cooking Instructions:

1. Spread peanut butter onto celery sticks for a crunchy and satisfying snack.

Day 12

Breakfast: **Berry Banana Smoothie Bowl**

Ingredients:

- 1 ripe banana, frozen

- 1/2 cup mixed berries (such as strawberries, blueberries, raspberries)

- 1/2 cup Greek yogurt

- 1/4 cup almond milk

- **Toppings:** sliced banana, fresh berries, granola, shredded coconut

Servings: 1

Prep Time: 5 minutes

Cooking Instructions:

1. In a blender, combine frozen banana, mixed berries, Greek yogurt, and almond milk.

2. Blend until smooth and creamy, adding more almond milk if needed to reach desired consistency.

3. Pour the smoothie into a bowl.

4. Top with sliced banana, fresh berries, granola, and shredded coconut.

5. Serve immediately with a spoon.

Lunch: **Mediterranean Chickpea Wrap**

Ingredients:

- 1 whole grain wrap or tortilla

- 1/2 cup canned chickpeas, rinsed and drained

- 1/4 cup diced cucumber

- 1/4 cup diced tomatoes

- 2 tablespoons crumbled feta cheese

- 2 tablespoons hummus

- Fresh parsley, chopped

Servings: 1

Prep Time: 10 minutes

Cooking Instructions:

1. Lay the whole grain wrap or tortilla on a flat surface.

2. Spread hummus evenly over the wrap.

3. In the center of the wrap, layer chickpeas, diced cucumber, diced tomatoes, crumbled feta

cheese, and chopped fresh parsley.

4. Fold in the sides of the wrap and roll it up tightly.

5. Slice the wrap in half diagonally if desired.

6. Serve immediately or wrap in foil for later.

Dinner: Teriyaki Tofu Stir-Fry

Ingredients:

- 1 block firm tofu, pressed and cubed

- 2 cups mixed vegetables (such as bell peppers, broccoli, snap peas, carrots)

- 2 cloves garlic, minced

- 1/4 cup low-sodium soy sauce

- 2 tablespoons honey or maple syrup

- 1 tablespoon rice vinegar

- 1 tablespoon cornstarch

- 1 tablespoon water

- Cooked brown rice for serving

Servings: 2

Prep Time: 15 minutes

Cooking Instructions:

1. In a small bowl, whisk together low-sodium soy sauce, honey or maple syrup, and rice vinegar to make the teriyaki sauce.

2. In another small bowl, mix cornstarch and water to make a slurry.

3. Heat a large skillet or wok over medium-high heat.

4. Add cubed tofu to the skillet and cook until golden brown on all sides.

5. Remove tofu from the skillet and set aside.

6. In the same skillet, add minced garlic and mixed vegetables. Stir-fry until vegetables are tender-crisp.

7. Return tofu to the skillet and pour the teriyaki sauce over the tofu and vegetables.

8. Stir in the cornstarch slurry and cook for another 2-3 minutes, or until the sauce has thickened.

9. Serve teriyaki tofu stir-fry over cooked brown rice.

Snack: Apple Slices with Cinnamon

Ingredients:

- 1 apple, sliced

- Cinnamon

Servings: 1

Prep Time: 2 minutes

Cooking Instructions:

1. Sprinkle apple slices with cinnamon for a simple and delicious snack.

Day 13

Breakfast: Veggie Breakfast Burrito

Ingredients:

- 1 whole wheat tortilla

- 2 eggs, scrambled

- 1/4 cup black beans, drained and rinsed

- 2 tablespoons diced bell peppers

- 2 tablespoons diced tomatoes

- 2 tablespoons diced onions

- 2 tablespoons shredded cheese

- Salsa and avocado slices for topping (optional)

Servings: 1

Prep Time: 10 minutes

- Cooking Instructions:

1. Heat a skillet over medium heat and spray with cooking spray.

2. Add diced onions and bell peppers to the skillet and sauté until softened.

3. Add scrambled eggs to the skillet and cook until set.

4. Warm the black beans in the skillet.

5. Place the tortilla on a plate and layer scrambled eggs, black beans, diced tomatoes, shredded cheese, salsa, and avocado slices.

6. Roll up the tortilla to form a burrito.

7. Serve immediately.

Lunch: Greek Chickpea Salad

Ingredients:

- 1 can chickpeas, rinsed and drained

- 1 cucumber, diced

- 1 cup cherry tomatoes, halved

- 1/4 cup diced red onion

- 1/4 cup Kalamata olives, pitted and sliced

- 2 tablespoons crumbled feta cheese

- 2 tablespoons chopped fresh parsley

- Juice of 1 lemon

- 2 tablespoons olive oil

- Salt and pepper to taste

Servings: 2

Prep Time: 10 minutes

Cooking Instructions:

1. In a large bowl, combine chickpeas, diced cucumber, cherry tomatoes, diced red onion, sliced Kalamata olives, crumbled feta cheese, and chopped fresh parsley.

2. In a small bowl, whisk together lemon juice, olive oil, salt, and pepper to make the dressing.

3. Pour the dressing over the chickpea salad and toss to coat evenly.

4. Serve chilled or at room temperature.

Dinner: Lemon Herb Grilled Salmon

Ingredients:

- 2 salmon fillets

- 2 tablespoons olive oil

- Zest and juice of 1 lemon

- 1 teaspoon dried thyme

- 1 teaspoon dried oregano

- Salt and pepper to taste

Servings: 2

Prep Time: 10 minutes

Cooking Instructions:

1. In a small bowl, whisk together olive oil, lemon zest, lemon juice, dried thyme, dried oregano, salt, and pepper.

2. Place salmon fillets in a shallow dish and pour the marinade over them, turning to coat evenly.

3. Cover and refrigerate for at least 30 minutes, or up to 1 hour.

4. Preheat the grill to medium-high heat.

5. Remove salmon from marinade and discard excess marinade.

6. Grill salmon for 4-5 minutes per side, or until fish flakes easily with a fork and is cooked to your desired doneness.

7. Serve hot.

Snack: Yogurt and Granola Parfait

Ingredients:

- 1 cup Greek yogurt

- 1/4 cup granola

- 1/4 cup mixed berries (such as strawberries, blueberries, raspberries)

Servings: 1

Prep Time: 2 minutes

Cooking Instructions:

1. In a glass or bowl, layer Greek yogurt, granola, and mixed berries.

2. Repeat layering if desired.

3. Serve immediately.

Day 14

Breakfast: Spinach and Mushroom Breakfast Quesadilla

Ingredients:

- 2 whole wheat tortillas

- 1/2 cup shredded cheese (such as cheddar or Monterey Jack)

- 1 cup baby spinach leaves

- 1/2 cup sliced mushrooms

- Cooking spray or olive oil

Servings: 1

Prep Time: 10 minutes

Cooking Instructions:

1. Heat a skillet over medium heat and spray with cooking spray or add a little olive oil.

2. Place one tortilla in the skillet and sprinkle half of the shredded cheese over it.

3. Layer baby spinach leaves and sliced mushrooms over the cheese.

4. Sprinkle the remaining shredded cheese over the spinach and mushrooms.

5. Top with the second tortilla.

6. Cook for 2-3 minutes on each side, or until the tortilla is golden brown and the cheese is melted.

7. Remove from the skillet and slice into wedges.

8. Serve hot.

Lunch: **Mediterranean Hummus Wrap**

Ingredients:

- 1 whole grain wrap or tortilla

- 2 tablespoons hummus

- 1/4 cup diced cucumber

- 1/4 cup diced tomatoes

- 1/4 cup sliced black olives

- 2 tablespoons crumbled feta cheese

- Fresh parsley, chopped

Servings: 1

Prep Time: 5 minutes

Cooking Instructions:

1. Spread hummus evenly over the whole grain wrap or tortilla.

2. Layer diced cucumber, diced tomatoes, sliced black olives, crumbled feta cheese, and chopped fresh parsley on top of the hummus.

3. Roll up the wrap tightly.

4. Slice in half diagonally if desired.

5. Serve immediately or wrap in foil for later.

Dinner: **Chicken and Vegetable Stir-Fry**

Ingredients:

- 2 boneless, skinless chicken breasts, thinly sliced

- 2 cups mixed vegetables (such as bell peppers, broccoli, snap peas, carrots)

- 2 cloves garlic, minced

- 2 tablespoons low-sodium soy sauce

- 1 tablespoon hoisin sauce

- 1 tablespoon sesame oil

- Cooked brown rice for serving

Servings: 2

Prep Time: 15 minutes

Cooking Instructions:

1. Heat sesame oil in a large skillet or wok over medium-high heat.

2. Add minced garlic to the skillet and sauté for 1 minute.

3. Add sliced chicken breasts to the skillet and cook until browned and cooked through.

4. Remove chicken from the skillet and set aside.

5. In the same skillet, add mixed vegetables and stir-fry until they are tender-crisp.

6. Return cooked chicken to the skillet.

7. In a small bowl, mix together low-sodium soy sauce and hoisin sauce. Pour over the chicken and vegetables.

8. Cook for another 2-3 minutes, stirring constantly, until everything is coated in the sauce.

9. Serve chicken and vegetable stir-fry over cooked brown rice.

Snack: Cottage Cheese with Pineapple

Ingredients:

- 1/2 cup cottage cheese

- 1/2 cup diced pineapple

Servings: 1

Prep Time: 2 minutes

Cooking Instructions:

1. Mix cottage cheese with diced pineapple for a creamy and sweet snack.

Day 15

Breakfast: Avocado Toast with Poached Egg

Ingredients:

- 2 slices whole grain bread, toasted

- 1 ripe avocado

- 2 eggs

- Salt and pepper to taste

Servings: 1

Prep Time: 10 minutes

- Cooking Instructions:

1. Mash the ripe avocado in a bowl and season with salt and pepper to taste.

2. Poach the eggs to your desired level of doneness.

3. Spread mashed avocado evenly onto the toasted whole grain bread slices.

4. Top each slice with a poached egg.

5. Sprinkle with additional salt and pepper if desired.

6. Serve immediately.

Lunch: Quinoa Salad with Roasted Vegetables

Ingredients:

- 1 cup cooked quinoa

- 2 cups mixed roasted vegetables (such as bell peppers, zucchini, eggplant, cherry tomatoes)

- 1/4 cup crumbled feta cheese

- 2 tablespoons chopped fresh parsley

- 2 tablespoons balsamic vinaigrette

Servings: 2

Prep Time: 15 minutes

Cooking Instructions:

1. In a large bowl, combine cooked quinoa, mixed roasted vegetables, crumbled feta cheese, and chopped fresh parsley.

2. Drizzle balsamic vinaigrette over the quinoa salad and toss to coat evenly.

3. Serve chilled or at room temperature.

Dinner: Lentil and Vegetable Curry

Ingredients:

- 1 cup dried lentils, rinsed

- 2 cups vegetable broth

- 1 onion, chopped

- 2 cloves garlic, minced

- 1 tablespoon curry powder

- 1 teaspoon ground cumin

- 1 teaspoon ground coriander

- 1/2 teaspoon turmeric

- 2 cups mixed vegetables (such as cauliflower, carrots, peas)

- 1 can (14 oz) diced tomatoes

- Salt and pepper to taste

Servings: 4

Prep Time: 10 minutes

Cooking Instructions:

1. In a large pot, combine dried lentils, vegetable broth, chopped onion, minced garlic, curry powder, ground cumin, ground coriander, and turmeric.

2. Bring to a boil, then reduce heat to low and simmer for 20-25 minutes, or until lentils are tender.

3. Add mixed vegetables and diced tomatoes to the pot.

4. Continue to simmer for another 10-15 minutes, or until vegetables are cooked through.

5. Season with salt and pepper to taste.

6. Serve hot, optionally with cooked rice or naan bread.

Snack: Trail Mix

Ingredients:

- 1/4 cup almonds

- 1/4 cup cashews

- 1/4 cup dried cranberries

- 1/4 cup dark chocolate chips

- Servings: 1

Prep Time: 2 minutes

Cooking Instructions:

1. Mix almonds, cashews, dried cranberries, and dark chocolate chips together to make a tasty trail mix.

Day 16

Breakfast: Berry Chia Seed Pudding

Ingredients:

- 1/4 cup chia seeds

- 1 cup almond milk

- 1/2 teaspoon vanilla extract

- 1/2 cup mixed berries (such as strawberries, blueberries, raspberries)

- Honey or maple syrup for sweetness (optional)

Servings: 1

Prep Time: 5 minutes (plus chilling time)

Cooking Instructions:

1. In a bowl or jar, mix together chia seeds, almond milk, and vanilla extract.

2. Stir in mixed berries.

3. Optionally, add honey or maple syrup for sweetness to taste.

4. Cover and refrigerate for at least 2 hours or overnight, until the chia pudding thickens.

5. Stir before serving and enjoy cold.

Lunch: Grilled Vegetable Panini

Ingredients:

- 4 slices whole grain bread

- 1 zucchini, thinly sliced lengthwise

- 1 yellow squash, thinly sliced lengthwise

- 1 red bell pepper, sliced into strips

- 1/4 cup pesto sauce

- 1/2 cup baby spinach leaves

- 1/4 cup crumbled feta cheese

- Olive oil for brushing

Servings: 2

Prep Time: 15 minutes

Cooking Instructions:

1. Preheat a grill pan or panini press.

2. Brush zucchini, yellow squash, and red bell pepper slices with olive oil.

3. Grill the vegetables until tender and grill marks appear, about 2-3 minutes per side.

4. Spread pesto sauce on one side of each slice of bread.

5. Layer grilled vegetables, baby spinach leaves, and crumbled feta cheese on two slices of bread.

6. Top with the remaining slices of bread to make sandwiches.

7. Grill the sandwiches in the panini press or grill pan until

golden brown and the cheese is melted, about 3-4 minutes.

8. Slice in half and serve hot.

Dinner: Baked Teriyaki Salmon

Ingredients:

- 2 salmon fillets

- 1/4 cup low-sodium soy sauce

- 2 tablespoons honey

- 1 tablespoon rice vinegar

- 1 clove garlic, minced

- 1 teaspoon grated ginger

- Sesame seeds for garnish (optional)

Servings: 2

Prep Time: 10 minutes

Cooking Instructions:

1. Preheat the oven to 400°F (200°C).

2. In a small bowl, whisk together low-sodium soy sauce, honey, rice vinegar, minced garlic, and grated ginger to make the teriyaki sauce.

3. Place salmon fillets in a baking dish and pour the teriyaki sauce over them, turning to coat evenly.

4. Bake in the preheated oven for 12-15 minutes, or until salmon is cooked through and flakes easily with a fork.

5. Remove from the oven and sprinkle with sesame seeds if desired.

6. Serve hot.

Snack: Greek Yogurt with Honey and Almonds

Ingredients:

- 1/2 cup Greek yogurt

- 1 tablespoon honey

- 2 tablespoons sliced almonds

Servings: 1

Prep Time: 2 minutes

Cooking Instructions:

1. Top Greek yogurt with honey and sliced almonds for a protein-rich and satisfying snack.

Day 17

Breakfast:

Ingredients:

- 1 whole wheat tortilla

- 2 eggs, scrambled

- 1/4 cup black beans, drained and rinsed

- 2 tablespoons diced bell peppers

- 2 tablespoons diced tomatoes

- 2 tablespoons diced onions

- 2 tablespoons shredded cheese

- Salsa and avocado slices for topping (optional)

Servings: 1

Prep Time: 10 minutes

Cooking Instructions:

1. Heat a skillet over medium heat and spray with cooking spray.

2. Add diced onions and bell peppers to the skillet and sauté until softened.

3. Add scrambled eggs to the skillet and cook until set.

4. Warm the black beans in the skillet.

5. Place the tortilla on a plate and layer scrambled eggs, black beans, diced tomatoes, shredded cheese, salsa, and avocado slices.

6. Roll up the tortilla to form a burrito.

7. Serve immediately.

Lunch: Greek Chickpea Salad

Ingredients:

- 1 can chickpeas, rinsed and drained

- 1 cucumber, diced

- 1 cup cherry tomatoes, halved

- 1/4 cup diced red onion

- 1/4 cup Kalamata olives, pitted and sliced

- 2 tablespoons crumbled feta cheese

- 2 tablespoons chopped fresh parsley

- Juice of 1 lemon

- 2 tablespoons olive oil

- Salt and pepper to taste

Servings: 2

Prep Time: 10 minutes

Cooking Instructions:

1. In a large bowl, combine chickpeas, diced cucumber, cherry tomatoes, diced red onion, sliced Kalamata olives, crumbled feta cheese, and chopped fresh parsley.

2. In a small bowl, whisk together lemon juice, olive oil, salt, and pepper to make the dressing.

3. Pour the dressing over the chickpea salad and toss to coat evenly.

4. Serve chilled or at room temperature.

Dinner: Lentil and Vegetable Curry

- Ingredients:

- 1 cup dried lentils, rinsed

- 2 cups vegetable broth

- 1 onion, chopped

- 2 cloves garlic, minced

- 1 tablespoon curry powder

- 1 teaspoon ground cumin

- 1 teaspoon ground coriander

- 1/2 teaspoon turmeric

- 2 cups mixed vegetables (such as cauliflower, carrots, peas)

- 1 can (14 oz) diced tomatoes

- Salt and pepper to taste

Servings: 4

Prep Time: 10 minutes

Cooking Instructions:

1. In a large pot, combine dried lentils, vegetable broth, chopped onion, minced garlic, curry powder, ground cumin, ground coriander, and turmeric.

2. Bring to a boil, then reduce heat to low and simmer for 20-25 minutes, or until lentils are tender.

3. Add mixed vegetables and diced tomatoes to the pot.

4. Continue to simmer for another 10-15 minutes, or until vegetables are cooked through.

5. Season with salt and pepper to taste.

6. Serve hot, optionally with cooked rice or naan bread.

Snack: Trail Mix

Ingredients:

- 1/4 cup almonds

- 1/4 cup cashews

- 1/4 cup dried cranberries

- 1/4 cup dark chocolate chips

- Servings: 1

- Prep Time: 2 minutes

- Cooking Instructions:

1. Mix almonds, cashews, dried cranberries, and dark chocolate chips together to make a tasty trail mix.

Day 18

Breakfast: Blueberry Banana Smoothie

- Ingredients:

- 1 ripe banana

- 1/2 cup blueberries (fresh or frozen)

- 1/2 cup spinach leaves

- 1/2 cup Greek yogurt

- 1/2 cup almond milk (or any milk of choice)

- 1 tablespoon honey or maple syrup (optional)

Servings: 1

Prep Time: 5 minutes

Cooking Instructions:

1. In a blender, combine banana, blueberries, spinach leaves, Greek yogurt, almond milk, and honey or maple syrup if using.

2. Blend until smooth and creamy.

3. Pour into a glass and serve immediately.

Lunch: Caprese Salad

Ingredients:

- 2 ripe tomatoes, sliced

- 1 ball fresh mozzarella cheese, sliced

- 1/4 cup fresh basil leaves

- 2 tablespoons balsamic glaze

- Salt and pepper to taste

Servings: 2

Prep Time: 5 minutes

Cooking Instructions:

1. Arrange tomato slices and mozzarella slices alternately on a serving plate.

2. Tuck fresh basil leaves in between the tomato and mozzarella slices.

3. Drizzle with balsamic glaze.

4. Season with salt and pepper to taste.

5. Serve immediately as a refreshing salad.

Dinner: Spaghetti Aglio e Olio with Shrimp

Ingredients:

- 8 oz spaghetti

- 2 tablespoons olive oil

- 4 cloves garlic, thinly sliced

- 1/4 teaspoon red pepper flakes

- 8 oz shrimp, peeled and deveined

- Salt and pepper to taste

- Fresh parsley, chopped

Servings: 2

Prep Time: 10 minutes

Cooking Instructions:

1. Cook spaghetti according to package instructions until al dente. Drain and set aside.

2. Heat olive oil in a large skillet over medium heat.

3. Add thinly sliced garlic and red pepper flakes to the skillet. Sauté until garlic is golden brown and fragrant.

4. Add shrimp to the skillet and cook until pink and opaque, about 2-3 minutes per side.

5. Season with salt and pepper to taste.

6. Add cooked spaghetti to the skillet and toss to coat with the garlic-infused oil.

7. Cook for another minute, allowing the flavors to meld together.

8. Sprinkle chopped fresh parsley over the spaghetti and shrimp before serving.

9. Serve hot.

Snack: Apple with Peanut Butter

Ingredients:

- 1 apple, sliced

- Peanut butter for dipping

Servings: 1

Prep Time: 2 minutes

Cooking Instructions:

1. Slice the apple and serve with peanut butter for dipping.

Day 19

Breakfast: Veggie Breakfast Scramble

Ingredients:

- 2 eggs

- 1/4 cup diced bell peppers

- 1/4 cup diced tomatoes

- 1/4 cup diced onions

- 1/4 cup spinach leaves

- Salt and pepper to taste

- Cooking spray or olive oil

Servings: 1

Prep Time: 10 minutes

Cooking Instructions:

1. Heat a non-stick skillet over medium heat and lightly coat with cooking spray or olive oil.

2. Add diced onions and bell peppers to the skillet and sauté until softened.

3. Add diced tomatoes and spinach leaves to the skillet and cook until spinach is wilted.

4. In a bowl, beat the eggs and season with salt and pepper.

5. Pour the beaten eggs into the skillet with the vegetables.

6. Cook, stirring occasionally, until eggs are set.

7. Serve hot.

Lunch: Quinoa Salad with Avocado

Ingredients:

- 1 cup cooked quinoa

- 1 ripe avocado, diced

- 1/2 cup cherry tomatoes, halved

- 1/4 cup diced cucumber

- 1/4 cup diced red onion

- 2 tablespoons chopped fresh cilantro

- Juice of 1 lime

- Salt and pepper to taste

Servings: 2

Prep Time: 10 minutes

Cooking Instructions:

1. In a large bowl, combine cooked quinoa, diced avocado, cherry tomatoes, diced cucumber, diced red onion, and chopped fresh cilantro.

2. Squeeze lime juice over the salad and toss to combine.

3. Season with salt and pepper to taste.

4. Serve chilled or at room temperature.

Dinner: Lemon Herb Grilled Chicken

Ingredients:

- 2 boneless, skinless chicken breasts

- 2 tablespoons olive oil

- Zest and juice of 1 lemon

- 2 cloves garlic, minced

- 1 teaspoon dried thyme

- 1 teaspoon dried rosemary

- Salt and pepper to taste

Servings: 2

Prep Time: 10 minutes

Cooking Instructions:

1. In a small bowl, whisk together olive oil, lemon zest, lemon juice, minced garlic, dried thyme, dried rosemary, salt, and pepper.

2. Place chicken breasts in a shallow dish and pour the marinade over them, turning to coat evenly.

3. Cover and refrigerate for at least 30 minutes, or up to 2 hours.

4. Preheat the grill to medium-high heat.

5. Remove chicken from marinade and discard excess marinade.

6. Grill chicken for 6-8 minutes per side, or until cooked through and no longer pink in the center.

7. Let chicken rest for a few minutes before serving.

8. Serve hot.

Snack: Greek Yogurt with Berries

Ingredients:

- 1/2 cup Greek yogurt

- 1/4 cup mixed berries (such as strawberries, blueberries, raspberries)

- Honey or maple syrup for sweetness (optional)

Servings: 1

Prep Time: 2 minutes

Cooking Instructions:

1. Top Greek yogurt with mixed berries.

2. Optionally, drizzle with honey or maple syrup for sweetness.

3. Serve chilled.

Day 20

Breakfast: Banana Nut Overnight Oats

Ingredients:

- 1/2 cup rolled oats

- 1/2 cup almond milk (or any milk of choice)

- 1/2 ripe banana, mashed

- 1 tablespoon chia seeds

- 1 tablespoon chopped walnuts

- 1/2 teaspoon vanilla extract

Servings: 1

Prep Time: 5 minutes (plus overnight chilling)

Cooking Instructions:

1. In a jar or container with a lid, combine rolled oats, almond milk, mashed banana, chia seeds, chopped walnuts, and vanilla extract.

2. Stir well to combine all ingredients.

3. Cover and refrigerate overnight, or for at least 4 hours.

4. In the morning, give the mixture a good stir and add more almond milk if desired for consistency.

5. Serve cold.

Lunch: Chickpea and Avocado Salad

Ingredients:

- 1 can chickpeas, rinsed and drained

- 1 ripe avocado, diced

- 1/2 cup cherry tomatoes, halved

- 1/4 cup diced cucumber

- 1/4 cup diced red onion

- 2 tablespoons chopped fresh parsley

- Juice of 1 lemon

- 2 tablespoons olive oil

- Salt and pepper to taste

Servings: 2

Prep Time: 10 minutes

Cooking Instructions:

1. In a large bowl, combine chickpeas, diced avocado, cherry tomatoes, diced cucumber, diced red onion, and chopped fresh parsley.

2. In a small bowl, whisk together lemon juice, olive oil, salt, and pepper to make the dressing.

3. Pour the dressing over the chickpea and avocado salad and toss to coat evenly.

4. Serve chilled or at room temperature.

Dinner: Baked Pesto Salmon

Ingredients:

- 2 salmon fillets

- 2 tablespoons pesto sauce

- 1 tablespoon lemon juice

- Salt and pepper to taste

Servings: 2

Prep Time: 5 minutes

Cooking Instructions:

1. Preheat the oven to 375°F (190°C).

2. Place salmon fillets on a

baking sheet lined with parchment paper.

3. Spread pesto sauce evenly over the salmon fillets.

4. Drizzle lemon juice over the salmon.

5. Season with salt and pepper to taste.

6. Bake in the preheated oven for 12-15 minutes, or until salmon is cooked through and flakes easily with a fork.

7. Serve hot.

Snack: **Carrot Sticks with Hummus**

- Ingredients:

- 1 carrot, peeled and cut into sticks

- Hummus for dipping

Servings: 1

Prep Time: 2 minutes

Cooking Instructions:

1. Serve carrot sticks with hummus for dipping.

Day 21

Breakfast: **Spinach and Feta Omelette**

Ingredients:

- 2 eggs

- 1/4 cup chopped spinach

- 2 tablespoons crumbled feta cheese

- Salt and pepper to taste

- Cooking spray or olive oil

Servings: 1

Prep Time: 5 minutes

Cooking Instructions:

1. In a bowl, beat the eggs and season with salt and pepper.

2. Heat a non-stick skillet over medium heat and lightly coat with cooking spray or olive oil.

3. Pour the beaten eggs into the skillet and tilt to spread evenly.

4. Cook for 2-3 minutes, or until the edges start to set.

5. Sprinkle chopped spinach and crumbled feta cheese over one half of the omelette.

6. Fold the other half of the omelette over the filling.

7. Cook for another 1-2 minutes, or until the cheese is melted and the omelette is cooked through.

8. Slide the omelette onto a plate and serve hot.

Lunch: Mediterranean Quinoa Bowl

- Ingredients:

- 1 cup cooked quinoa

- 1/4 cup diced cucumber

- 1/4 cup diced tomatoes

- 1/4 cup sliced Kalamata olives

- 2 tablespoons crumbled feta cheese

- 2 tablespoons chopped fresh parsley

- 1 tablespoon lemon juice

- 1 tablespoon olive oil

- Salt and pepper to taste

Servings: 1

Prep Time: 10 minutes

Cooking Instructions:

1. In a bowl, combine cooked quinoa, diced cucumber, diced tomatoes, sliced Kalamata olives, crumbled feta cheese, and chopped fresh parsley.

2. In a small bowl, whisk together lemon juice, olive oil, salt, and pepper to make the dressing.

3. Pour the dressing over the quinoa bowl and toss to coat evenly.

4. Serve chilled or at room temperature.

Dinner: Teriyaki Tofu Stir-Fry

Ingredients:

- 8 oz extra-firm tofu, pressed and cubed

- 2 tablespoons low-sodium soy sauce

- 1 tablespoon hoisin sauce

- 1 tablespoon rice vinegar

- 1 clove garlic, minced

- 1 teaspoon grated ginger

- 1 tablespoon sesame oil

- 2 cups mixed vegetables (such as bell peppers, broccoli, snap peas, carrots)

- Cooked brown rice for serving

Servings: 2

Prep Time: 15 minutes

Cooking Instructions:

1. In a bowl, combine cubed tofu, low-sodium soy sauce, hoisin sauce, rice vinegar, minced garlic, and grated ginger. Allow to marinate for 10-15 minutes.

2. Heat sesame oil in a large skillet or wok over medium-high heat.

3. Add marinated tofu to the skillet and cook until browned on all sides.

4. Remove tofu from the skillet and set aside.

5. In the same skillet, add mixed vegetables and stir-fry until they are tender-crisp.

6. Return cooked tofu to the skillet.

7. Cook for another 2-3 minutes, stirring constantly.

8. Serve tofu and vegetable stir-fry over cooked brown rice.

Snack: Cottage Cheese with Pineapple

Ingredients:

- 1/2 cup cottage cheese

- 1/2 cup diced pineapple

Servings: 1

Prep Time: 2 minutes

Cooking Instructions:

1. Mix cottage cheese with diced pineapple for a protein-rich and refreshing snack.

Day 22

Breakfast: Berry Protein Smoothie

- Ingredients:

  - 1/2 cup mixed berries (such as strawberries, blueberries, raspberries)

  - 1/2 banana

  - 1/2 cup Greek yogurt

  - 1/2 cup almond milk (or any milk of choice)

  - 1 scoop protein powder (optional)

Servings: 1

Prep Time: 5 minutes

Cooking Instructions:

  1. In a blender, combine mixed berries, banana, Greek yogurt, almond milk, and protein powder if using.

  2. Blend until smooth and creamy.

  3. Add more almond milk if needed to reach desired consistency.

  4. Serve immediately.

Lunch: Mediterranean Chickpea Salad

Ingredients:

  - 1 can chickpeas, rinsed and drained

  - 1/2 cucumber, diced

  - 1/2 cup cherry tomatoes, halved

  - 1/4 cup diced red onion

  - 1/4 cup sliced Kalamata olives

  - 2 tablespoons chopped fresh parsley

  - 2 tablespoons crumbled feta cheese

  - Juice of 1 lemon

  - 2 tablespoons olive oil

  - Salt and pepper to taste

Servings: 2

Prep Time: 10 minutes

Cooking Instructions:

  1. In a large bowl, combine chickpeas, diced cucumber, cherry tomatoes, diced red onion, sliced Kalamata olives, chopped fresh parsley, and crumbled feta cheese.

2. In a small bowl, whisk together lemon juice, olive oil, salt, and pepper to make the dressing.

3. Pour the dressing over the chickpea salad and toss to coat evenly.

4. Serve chilled or at room temperature.

Dinner: Grilled Lemon Herb Chicken with Roasted Vegetables

Ingredients:

- 2 boneless, skinless chicken breasts

- Zest and juice of 1 lemon

- 2 cloves garlic, minced

- 1 teaspoon dried thyme

- 1 teaspoon dried rosemary

- Salt and pepper to taste

- 2 cups mixed vegetables (such as bell peppers, zucchini, carrots)

- 1 tablespoon olive oil

Servings: 2

Prep Time: 15 minutes

Cooking Instructions:

1. In a bowl, combine lemon zest, lemon juice, minced garlic, dried thyme, dried rosemary, salt, and pepper.

2. Place chicken breasts in a shallow dish and pour the marinade over them, turning to coat evenly.

3. Cover and refrigerate for at least 30 minutes, or up to 2 hours.

4. Preheat the grill to medium-high heat.

5. Remove chicken from marinade and discard excess marinade.

6. Grill chicken for 6-8 minutes per side, or until cooked through and no longer pink in the center.

7. Meanwhile, toss mixed vegetables with olive oil, salt, and pepper.

8. Roast vegetables in the oven at 400°F (200°C) for 15-20 minutes, or until tender.

9. Serve grilled lemon herb chicken with roasted vegetables.

Snack: Apple Slices with Almond Butter

Ingredients:

- 1 apple, sliced

- Almond butter for dipping

Servings: 1

Prep Time: 2 minutes

Cooking Instructions:

1. Slice the apple and serve with almond butter for dipping.

Day 23

Breakfast: Veggie Breakfast Burrito

Ingredients:

- 1 whole wheat tortilla

- 2 eggs, scrambled

- 1/4 cup black beans, drained and rinsed

- 2 tablespoons diced bell peppers

- 2 tablespoons diced tomatoes

- 2 tablespoons diced onions

- 2 tablespoons shredded cheese

- Salsa and avocado slices for topping (optional)

Servings: 1

Prep Time: 10 minutes

Cooking Instructions:

1. Heat a skillet over medium heat and spray with cooking spray.

2. Add diced onions and bell peppers to the skillet and sauté until softened.

3. Add scrambled eggs to the skillet and cook until set.

4. Warm the black beans in the skillet.

5. Place the tortilla on a plate and layer scrambled eggs, black beans, diced tomatoes, shredded cheese, salsa, and avocado slices.

6. Roll up the tortilla to form a burrito.

7. Serve immediately.

Lunch: Greek Quinoa Salad

Ingredients:

- 1 cup cooked quinoa

- 1/2 cucumber, diced

- 1/2 cup cherry tomatoes, halved

- 1/4 cup diced red onion

- 1/4 cup Kalamata olives, pitted and sliced

- 2 tablespoons crumbled feta cheese

- 2 tablespoons chopped fresh parsley

- Juice of 1 lemon

- 2 tablespoons olive oil

- Salt and pepper to taste

Servings: 2

Prep Time: 10 minutes

Cooking Instructions:

1. In a large bowl, combine cooked quinoa, diced cucumber, cherry tomatoes, diced red onion, sliced Kalamata olives, crumbled feta cheese, and chopped fresh parsley.

2. In a small bowl, whisk together lemon juice, olive oil, salt, and pepper to make the dressing.

3. Pour the dressing over the quinoa salad and toss to coat evenly.

4. Serve chilled or at room temperature.

Dinner: Lemon Garlic Shrimp Pasta

Ingredients:

- 8 oz whole wheat spaghetti

- 8 oz shrimp, peeled and deveined

- 2 tablespoons olive oil

- 3 cloves garlic, minced

- Zest and juice of 1 lemon

- 1/4 teaspoon red pepper flakes

- Salt and pepper to taste

- Chopped fresh parsley for garnish

Servings: 2

Prep Time: 15 minutes

Cooking Instructions:

1. Cook spaghetti according to package instructions until al dente. Drain and set aside.

2. Heat olive oil in a large skillet over medium heat.

3. Add minced garlic and red pepper flakes to the skillet. Sauté until garlic is fragrant, about 1 minute.

4. Add shrimp to the skillet and cook until pink and opaque, about 2-3 minutes per side.

5. Stir in lemon zest and lemon juice.

6. Season with salt and pepper to taste.

7. Add cooked spaghetti to the skillet and toss to coat with the lemon garlic shrimp.

8. Garnish with chopped fresh parsley before serving.

9. Serve hot.

Snack: Greek Yogurt with Honey and Almonds

Ingredients:

- 1/2 cup Greek yogurt

- 1 tablespoon honey

- 2 tablespoons sliced almonds

Servings: 1

Prep Time: 2 minutes

Cooking Instructions:

1. Top Greek yogurt with honey and sliced almonds for a protein-rich and satisfying snack.

Day 24

Breakfast: Spinach and Mushroom Frittata

Ingredients:

- 4 eggs

- 1 cup fresh spinach, chopped

- 1/2 cup mushrooms, sliced

- 1/4 cup diced onion

- 1/4 cup shredded cheese (such as cheddar or mozzarella)

- Salt and pepper to taste

- Cooking spray or olive oil

Servings: 2

Prep Time: 10 minutes

Cooking Instructions:

1. Preheat the oven to 350°F (175°C).

2. In a bowl, beat the eggs and season with salt and pepper.

3. Heat an oven-safe skillet over medium heat and lightly coat with cooking spray or olive oil.

4. Add diced onion and sliced mushrooms to the skillet and sauté until softened.

5. Add chopped spinach to the skillet and cook until wilted.

6. Pour the beaten eggs over the vegetables in the skillet.

7. Sprinkle shredded cheese evenly over the eggs and vegetables.

8. Transfer the skillet to the preheated oven and bake for 10-12 minutes, or until the eggs are set and the cheese is melted and bubbly.

9. Slice into wedges and serve hot.

Lunch: Mediterranean Chickpea Wrap

Ingredients:

- 1 whole wheat wrap or tortilla

- 1/2 cup cooked chickpeas, mashed

- 1/4 cup diced cucumber

- 1/4 cup diced tomatoes

- 2 tablespoons diced red onion

- 2 tablespoons sliced Kalamata olives

- 2 tablespoons crumbled feta cheese

- 1 tablespoon chopped fresh parsley

- Juice of 1/2 lemon

- Salt and pepper to taste

Servings: 1

Prep Time: 10 minutes

Cooking Instructions:

1. In a bowl, combine mashed chickpeas, diced cucumber, diced tomatoes, diced red onion, sliced Kalamata olives, crumbled feta cheese, chopped fresh parsley, lemon juice, salt, and pepper.

2. Lay the whole wheat wrap or tortilla on a flat surface.

3. Spoon the chickpea mixture onto the center of the wrap.

4. Fold in the sides of the wrap and then roll it up tightly.

5. Slice in half if desired and serve.

Dinner: Turkey and Vegetable Stir-Fry

Ingredients:

- 8 oz turkey breast, thinly sliced

- 2 cups mixed vegetables (such as bell peppers, broccoli, snap peas, carrots)

- 2 tablespoons low-sodium soy sauce

- 1 tablespoon hoisin sauce

- 1 tablespoon sesame oil

- 2 cloves garlic, minced

- 1 teaspoon grated ginger

- 2 green onions, chopped

- Cooked brown rice for serving

Servings: 2

Prep Time: 15 minutes

Cooking Instructions:

1. Heat sesame oil in a large skillet or wok over medium-high heat.

2. Add minced garlic and grated ginger to the skillet. Sauté until fragrant, about 1 minute.

3. Add thinly sliced turkey breast to the skillet and cook until browned and cooked through.

4. Add mixed vegetables to the skillet and stir-fry until they are tender-crisp.

5. In a small bowl, mix together low-sodium soy sauce and hoisin sauce.

6. Pour the sauce over the turkey and vegetables in the skillet.

7. Stir well to coat everything evenly with the sauce.

8. Cook for another 2-3 minutes, or until heated through.

9. Garnish with chopped green onions before serving.

10. Serve turkey and vegetable stir-fry over cooked brown rice.

Snack: Celery Sticks with Peanut Butter

- Ingredients:

- Celery sticks

- Peanut butter for dipping

Servings: 1

Prep Time: 2 minutes

Cooking Instructions:

1. Serve celery sticks with peanut butter for dipping.

Day 25

Breakfast: **Berry Chia Seed Pudding**

- Ingredients:

  - 1/4 cup chia seeds

  - 1 cup almond milk (or any milk of choice)

  - 1/2 teaspoon vanilla extract

  - 1/2 cup mixed berries (such as strawberries, blueberries, raspberries)

  - 1 tablespoon honey or maple syrup (optional)

Servings: 1

Prep Time: 5 minutes (plus chilling time)

Cooking Instructions:

1. In a bowl or jar, mix together chia seeds, almond milk, and vanilla extract.

2. Stir in mixed berries and sweetener of choice if desired.

3. Cover and refrigerate for at least 2 hours, or overnight, until the chia seeds have absorbed the liquid and the mixture has thickened to a pudding-like consistency.

4. Stir well before serving.

Lunch: **Quinoa and Black Bean Salad**

Ingredients:

 - 1 cup cooked quinoa

 - 1/2 cup black beans, drained and rinsed

 - 1/2 cup corn kernels (fresh, canned, or frozen)

 - 1/4 cup diced bell peppers

 - 1/4 cup diced tomatoes

 - 2 tablespoons chopped fresh cilantro

 - Juice of 1 lime

- 1 tablespoon olive oil

- Salt and pepper to taste

Servings: 2

Prep Time: 10 minutes

Cooking Instructions:

1. In a large bowl, combine cooked quinoa, black beans, corn kernels, diced bell peppers, diced tomatoes, and chopped fresh cilantro.

2. In a small bowl, whisk together lime juice, olive oil, salt, and pepper to make the dressing.

3. Pour the dressing over the quinoa and black bean salad and toss to coat evenly.

4. Serve chilled or at room temperature.

Dinner: Salmon with Asparagus and Lemon Dill Sauce

Ingredients:

- 2 salmon fillets

- 1 bunch asparagus, trimmed

- 2 tablespoons olive oil

- Salt and pepper to taste

- Zest and juice of 1 lemon

- 2 tablespoons chopped fresh dill

Servings: 2

Prep Time: 10 minutes

Cooking Instructions:

1. Preheat the oven to 400°F (200°C).

2. Place salmon fillets on a baking sheet lined with parchment paper.

3. Arrange trimmed asparagus around the salmon on the baking sheet.

4. Drizzle olive oil over the salmon and asparagus.

5. Season salmon and asparagus with salt, pepper, lemon zest, and chopped fresh dill.

6. Squeeze lemon juice over the salmon.

7. Bake in the preheated oven for 12-15 minutes, or until the salmon is cooked through and flakes easily with a fork.

8. Serve hot.

Snack: Cucumber Slices with Hummus

Ingredients:

- 1 cucumber, sliced

- Hummus for dipping

Servings: 1

Prep Time: 2 minutes

Cooking Instructions:

1. Serve cucumber slices with hummus for dippin

Day 26

Breakfast: Avocado Toast with Poached Egg

Ingredients:

- 2 slices whole grain bread, toasted

- 1 ripe avocado, mashed

- 2 eggs

- Salt and pepper to taste

Servings: 2

Prep Time: 10 minutes

Cooking Instructions:

1. Poach the eggs: Bring a pot of water to a gentle simmer. Crack each egg into a small bowl or ramekin. Carefully slide the eggs into the simmering water. Poach for about 3-4 minutes until the whites are set but the yolks are still runny. Remove with a slotted spoon and drain excess water.

2. Spread mashed avocado evenly onto the toasted bread slices.

3. Place one poached egg on each slice of avocado toast.

4. Season with salt and pepper to taste.

5. Serve immediately.

Lunch: Chickpea and Avocado Wrap

Ingredients:

- 1 whole wheat wrap or tortilla

- 1/2 cup canned chickpeas, drained and rinsed

- 1/2 avocado, sliced

- 1/4 cup diced cucumber

- 1/4 cup diced tomatoes

- 2 tablespoons diced red onion

- 2 tablespoons chopped fresh cilantro

- Juice of 1/2 lime

- Salt and pepper to taste

Servings: 1

Prep Time: 10 minutes

Cooking Instructions:

1. In a bowl, mash the chickpeas with a fork until slightly chunky.

2. Add diced cucumber, diced tomatoes, diced red onion, chopped fresh cilantro, lime juice, salt, and pepper to the mashed chickpeas. Mix well.

3. Lay the whole wheat wrap or tortilla on a flat surface.

4. Spread the chickpea mixture onto the center of the wrap.

5. Top with sliced avocado.

6. Fold in the sides of the wrap and then roll it up tightly.

7. Slice in half if desired and serve.

Dinner: Turkey and Vegetable Skillet

Ingredients:

- 8 oz ground turkey

- 1 tablespoon olive oil

- 1/2 onion, diced

- 2 cloves garlic, minced

- 1 bell pepper, diced

- 1 zucchini, diced

- 1 cup cherry tomatoes, halved

- 1 teaspoon dried oregano

- 1 teaspoon dried basil

- Salt and pepper to taste

Servings: 2

Prep Time: 15 minutes

Cooking Instructions:

1. Heat olive oil in a large skillet over medium heat.

2. Add diced onion and minced garlic to the skillet. Sauté until softened and fragrant.

3. Add ground turkey to the skillet and cook until browned, breaking it apart with a spoon as it cooks.

4. Stir in diced bell pepper, diced zucchini, cherry tomatoes, dried oregano, and dried basil.

5. Cook until the vegetables are tender and the tomatoes have softened.

6. Season with salt and pepper to taste.

7. Serve hot.

Snack: Greek Yogurt Parfait

Ingredients:

- 1/2 cup Greek yogurt

- 1/4 cup granola

- 1/4 cup mixed berries (such as strawberries, blueberries, raspberries)

Servings: 1

Prep Time: 2 minutes

Cooking Instructions:

1. In a glass or bowl, layer Greek yogurt, granola, and mixed berries.

2. Repeat layers if desired.

3. Serve chilled.

Day 27

Breakfast: Banana Walnut Pancakes

Ingredients:

- 1 ripe banana, mashed

- 1 egg

- 1/4 cup almond milk (or any milk of choice)

- 1/2 cup whole wheat flour

- 1/2 teaspoon baking powder

- 1/4 teaspoon ground cinnamon

- 1/4 cup chopped walnuts

- Cooking spray or butter for greasing

- Maple syrup for serving (optional)

Servings: 2

Prep Time: 10 minutes

Cooking Instructions:

1. In a bowl, whisk together mashed banana, egg, and almond milk until well combined.

2. In another bowl, mix whole wheat flour, baking powder, and ground cinnamon.

3. Gradually add the dry ingredients to the wet ingredients, stirring until just combined.

4. Fold in chopped walnuts.

5. Heat a non-stick skillet or griddle over medium heat and lightly coat with cooking spray or butter.

6. Pour about 1/4 cup of batter onto the skillet for each pancake.

7. Cook until bubbles form on the surface of the pancake, then flip and cook until golden brown on the other side.

8. Repeat with the remaining batter.

9. Serve warm with maple syrup if desired.

Lunch: Veggie Wrap with Hummus

Ingredients:

- 1 whole wheat wrap or tortilla

- 2 tablespoons hummus

- 1/4 cup shredded carrots

- 1/4 cup shredded lettuce

- 1/4 cup sliced cucumber

- 1/4 cup diced bell peppers

- Salt and pepper to taste

Servings: 1

Prep Time: 5 minutes

Cooking Instructions:

1. Spread hummus evenly onto the whole wheat wrap or tortilla.

2. Layer shredded carrots, shredded lettuce, sliced cucumber, and diced bell peppers on top of the hummus.

3. Season with salt and pepper to taste.

4. Roll up the wrap tightly.

5. Slice in half if desired and serve.

Dinner: Lentil and Vegetable Stew

Ingredients:

- 1 tablespoon olive oil

- 1 onion, diced

- 2 cloves garlic, minced

- 2 carrots, diced

- 2 celery stalks, diced

- 1 cup dry green lentils, rinsed

- 4 cups vegetable broth

- 1 can (14 oz) diced tomatoes

- 1 teaspoon dried thyme

- 1 teaspoon dried oregano

- Salt and pepper to taste

Servings: 4

Prep Time: 10 minutes

Cooking Instructions:

1. Heat olive oil in a large pot over medium heat.

2. Add diced onion and minced garlic to the pot. Sauté until softened and fragrant.

3. Add diced carrots and celery to the pot and cook for a few minutes.

4. Stir in rinsed green lentils, vegetable broth, diced tomatoes (with their juices), dried thyme, and dried oregano.

5. Bring the mixture to a boil, then reduce heat to low and let simmer for about 25-30 minutes, or until the lentils are tender.

6. Season with salt and pepper to taste.

7. Serve hot.

Snack: Apple Slices with Peanut Butter

Ingredients:

- 1 apple, sliced

- Peanut butter for dipping

Servings: 1

Prep Time: 2 minutes

Cooking Instructions:

1. Serve apple slices with peanut butter for dipping.

Day 28

Breakfast: Blueberry Almond Smoothie Bowl

Ingredients:

- 1/2 cup frozen blueberries

- 1/2 banana

- 1/2 cup spinach

- 1/2 cup almond milk (or any milk of choice)

- 2 tablespoons almond butter

- 1 tablespoon chia seeds

- Toppings: sliced almonds, fresh blueberries, granola, honey (optional)

Servings: 1

Prep Time: 5 minutes

Cooking Instructions:

1. In a blender, combine frozen blueberries, banana, spinach, almond milk, almond butter, and chia seeds.

2. Blend until smooth and creamy.

3. Pour the smoothie into a bowl.

4. Top with sliced almonds, fresh blueberries, granola, and a drizzle of honey if desired.

5. Serve immediately.

Lunch: Caprese Salad

Ingredients:

- 1 large tomato, sliced

- 1 ball fresh mozzarella cheese, sliced

- Fresh basil leaves

- 1 tablespoon balsamic glaze

- Salt and pepper to taste

- Servings: 1

- Prep Time: 5 minutes

- Cooking Instructions:

1. Arrange tomato and mozzarella slices alternately on a plate.

2. Tuck fresh basil leaves between the tomato and mozzarella slices.

3. Drizzle balsamic glaze over the salad.

4. Season with salt and pepper to taste.

5. Serve immediately.

Dinner: Quinoa Stuffed Bell Peppers

Ingredients:

- 2 bell peppers, halved and seeds removed

- 1 cup cooked quinoa

- 1/2 cup black beans, drained and rinsed

- 1/2 cup corn kernels (fresh, canned, or frozen)

- 1/4 cup diced tomatoes

- 1/4 cup diced red onion

- 1/4 cup shredded cheese (such as cheddar or mozzarella)

- 1 teaspoon chili powder

- 1/2 teaspoon cumin

- Salt and pepper to taste

Servings: 2

Prep Time: 15 minutes

Cooking Instructions:

1. Preheat the oven to 375°F (190°C).

2. In a large bowl, mix together cooked quinoa, black beans, corn kernels, diced tomatoes, diced red onion, shredded cheese, chili powder, cumin, salt, and pepper.

3. Stuff each bell pepper half with the quinoa mixture.

4. Place stuffed bell peppers in a baking dish.

5. Cover the dish with foil and bake in the preheated oven for 25-30 minutes, or until the peppers are tender.

6. Remove the foil and bake for an additional 5 minutes, or until the cheese is melted and bubbly.

7. Serve hot.

Snack: Greek Yogurt with Berries

Ingredients:

- 1/2 cup Greek yogurt

- 1/4 cup mixed berries (such as strawberries, blueberries, raspberries)

- 1 tablespoon honey (optional)

Servings: 1

Prep Time: 2 minutes

Cooking Instructions:

1. In a bowl, layer Greek yogurt and mixed berries.

2. Drizzle with honey if desired.

3. Serve chilled.

Congratulations on completing the 28-day meal plan! You've made it to the end of your nutritious and delicious journey. Feel free to repeat any of your favorite recipes or explore new ones to maintain a healthy lifestyle.

CHAPTER 12

LIFESTYLE SUGGESTIONS FOR HEPATIC FUNCTION

Exercise's Effect On Liver Function

Exercise is essential for maintaining the health and function of the liver. One essential organ for many metabolic functions, including as detoxification and glucose management, is the liver. It has been demonstrated that regular exercise improves these processes, supporting a healthier liver.

Cardiovascular exercise, such as jogging, cycling, or brisk walking, increases the amount of blood flowing to the liver. The liver can digest nutrients and poisons more effectively because of the increased blood circulation. Exercise also helps with weight control and lowers the risk of non-alcoholic fatty liver disease (NAFLD), a disorder where fat builds up in the liver.

An additional component of exercise that supports liver function is resistance training. Increasing muscle mass can improve insulin sensitivity, which is necessary to keep blood sugar levels in check. Enhanced insulin sensitivity lowers the chance of developing liver-related disorders such as insulin resistance and type 2 diabetes.

Regular exercise also helps with weight control. A major risk factor for liver illnesses, such as cirrhosis and fatty liver disease, is obesity. Physical activity can help people maintain a healthy weight, which lowers their risk of liver-related problems.

Techniques for Stress Management

Liver health can be adversely affected by prolonged stress. Stress causes the body to release hormones like cortisol, which over time can lead to inflammation and liver damage. Using stress-reduction strategies that work is essential to keeping the liver healthy.

Stress can be decreased by engaging in mindfulness, meditation, and deep breathing techniques. These methods have a beneficial effect on the body's physiological reactions to stress in addition to calming the mind. Particularly yoga, which incorporates both physical exercise and mindfulness, has been demonstrated to support liver function by lowering inflammation and oxidative stress.

Creating a work-life balance is yet another crucial component of stress reduction. Extended work hours and ongoing stress can be associated with bad lifestyle choices, such as inadequate exercise and food that ultimately impact liver function. Making leisure and relaxation a priority can improve liver health and general well-being.

<u>Extra Lifestyle Modifications for a Healthy Liver</u>

Certain lifestyle modifications can enhance liver health in addition to physical activity and stress reduction. Keeping up a healthy, well-balanced diet is one important component. Eating meals high in antioxidants, like whole grains, fruits, and vegetables, can help shield the liver from oxidative damage.Alcohol use must be kept to a minimum for liver health. Cirrhosis and alcoholic liver disease are two disorders that can result from excessive alcohol use. For best liver function, follow suggested alcohol consumption guidelines or refrain from alcohol completely.Drinking enough of water is also essential. Water aids in the removal of toxins from the body, especially those the liver processes. Maintaining proper hydration facilitates the liver's detoxifying activities and guarantees peak performance.